THE AUTUMN
BRAIN SEMINARS

The Autumn Brain Seminars

Volume One

Edison K. Miyawaki, M.D.

To order additional copies of this book, contact:
Xlibris
844-714-8691
www.Xlibris.com
Orders@Xlibris.com
836994

CONTENTS

THIRD SEMINAR
Learning the Brainstem

Proposal

I envision four to six participants for a six-week period. The target audience would be those who've been exposed to introductory neuroanatomy. Yet they seek more. I write in 2021, still in the midst of a pandemic that started in 2019. No one knows the fate of the classroom as once we knew it.

Each week, there's a preliminary assignment, to read the first seminar, the second, and so forth. The reading only encourages each person to choose some aspect of that reading to explore *for the group*. Sessions, two-ish hours in length, happen once weekly. Thursdays in autumn before Boston's winter solstice would be best, in the afternoon, when the sun sets early anyway.

Everybody presents every week, save for one person. He, the seminar's organizer and author of this book in its two volumes, is present as a secretary for ideas raised.

*

All references are listed, per seminar, at the end of each volume. I apologize for some duplication of references across seminars, and I accept responsibility for all my errors of commission and omission.

These two autumn volumes incorporate revisions of six monographs previously published from 2018 to 2020. I have attempted to tighten the prose, to correct some obvious errors, and otherwise to improve on work that has occupied me during the latter part of my career.

The Crossed Organization of Brains

1

Left and Right

The student's question is: "The right brain controls the left body; the left brain, the right body. Why?"

Before we address why, is the statement correct? If one asked a non-medical person today, "what comes to mind when I say 'right brain'?" maybe the answer would be art, creativity, or something aside from control of the left body. Our student is in medical school, so she refers to knowledge we teach there–for example, that the cerebral cortex has to do with voluntary movement. To understand in what way the cerebral cortex and movement are related, we ask students to visualize or to draw a pyramidal tract (*tractus* in Latin refers to a drawing) starting, say, in the left frontal brain.

Axons arising from large pyramidal (Betz) neurons in the fifth layer of the left primary motor cortex, located anterior to the central sulcus, make up part–by no means all–of the fibers of the left internal capsule. Many, not all, left internal capsular fibers eventually form the left pyramid in the medulla, and the majority of those fibers will cross the midline–they'll decussate–in the low medulla to form a contralateral, right corticospinal tract in the spinal cord. To repeat, not all fibers of the pyramidal tract cross the midline in the low medulla, but most do. Interruptions of the tract on the left side above the decussation or on the right side below it will impair movement in the right hemibody. The pyramidal tract is an example of crossed organization in the brain. So: the left brain, we conclude with some rationality, *does* control movement in the right body.

Nevertheless, there are exceptions. Some tracts never cross the midline. Control of half of the body involves both crossed and uncrossed organizations.

What's an example of an uncrossed tract? Let's discuss just one. The vestibular system is also involved in the control of movement. We can draw a vestibulospinal tract, for example, in the right brain. (There's both a medial and a lateral vestibulospinal tract; neither crosses the midline. We'll concentrate on the lateral one.)

A vestibule, from the Latin, refers to some separate space, like a hotel lobby at a distance from your own room. The vestibular apparatus is located in an intricately hollowed cavity in the temporal bone at a distance from the brain and brainstem. As with other afferent inputs to brain, fibers carrying information from vestibular sensory epithelia have cell bodies in a ganglion—so-called Scarpa's ganglion, which is located inside the vestibular nerve itself.

Vestibular afferent fibers (from the right vestibule) innervate several vestibular nuclei in the right brainstem, but there's something unique about the lateral vestibular nucleus of Deiters, from whence fibers of the lateral vestibulospinal tract arise. The main afferents to the right, lateral vestibular nucleus are axons from Purkinje cells of the right, paramedian *vermis* of cerebellum. Then a right, lateral vestibulospinal tract originates in Deiters' nucleus and descends, without decussation, in the ventrolateral spinal cord as far as lumbar levels. It's a pathway which facilitates limb extension and inhibits limb flexion on the same side of the body.

Maybe the student wasn't worried so much about what the brain controls. The real curiosity had to do with the anatomical existence of crossroads. Without comment about the control of anything, let's concede that there are crossed and uncrossed pathways in all kinds of nervous systems. Reflex action in a nerve net, like a hydra's, has nothing to do with some decussation of fibers across the midline axis of a hydra. Likewise, if I tap a patellar tendon at a human knee, a normal reflex response has to do with neural connections only on one side of the body. One needn't talk about crossed tracts at all. Vertebrate nervous systems certainly have decussations, but contemporary studies of literally all the connections among the 300-odd neurons of *C. elegans* find that some projections cross the midline, some don't, but decussations occur even in that humble, invertebrate worm.

In medical school, we memorize the pathways relevant to the practice of human neurology. We commit to knowing some stolid facts–where specifically a pathway crosses the midline, and which pathways never cross. Then, to borrow Ramón y Cajal's lovely phrase, maybe we can think at long last about "the texture of the nervous system"–truly how it is woven, rather than ask why it is woven as it is.

All the same, the student's question is hard to avoid for anyone interested in the structure of brains.

2

A Problem with Teleologies

Over the next three chapters, in reverse chronological order of their publication dates, I'll discuss three papers whose arguments I found interesting and relevant to this first seminar. All have to do with what's been called the teleology of decussation. A word to the wise as we start: the telos—literally, the end—isn't known, because we haven't arrived there yet. When we think teleologically, we guess about the final, definitive purpose of something. But we really don't know the telos.

The strangest of the papers, by Kinsbourne from 2013, wrestles with an idea which he advanced first in the 1970's, although similar notions had been discussed as early as the 1820's. A major structural difference between a crayfish (an invertebrate) and a vertebrate has to do with where the neuraxis is located in relationship to the digestive tract. A cephalic swelling that we identify as the invertebrate brain, just like the vertebrate brain, lies dorsal to the oropharnyx and digestive tract, but the neuraxis (read: the rest of the contiguous nervous system) is ventral to the digestive tract in invertebrates.

We should pause a moment to visualize the schema fully. If I'm a crayfish, my brain is above and behind my mouth just as my human brain is, but my spinal cord passes to the front of me, anterior/ventral to my esophagus, stomach, and the rest of my bowels. But I am human—what follows applies to sharks and other chordates as well as all vertebrates–, so: my brain, spinal cord, and my spine (the notochord in a chordate) are all posterior/dorsal to my gut.

But: an obvious similarity between crayfish and humans is bilateral symmetry along the body's length. Evolutionists have long speculated about an ur-bilaterian creature whose axial symmetry anticipates all subsequent invertebrate, chordate, and vertebral body plans. Interspecies conservation of genes between vertebrates and invertebrates (like homeotic HOX genes in embryonic development) argues for the possibility of such a primordial common ancestor. At some point in the transition to the vertebrate nervous system and body, Kinsbourne maintains, maybe the brain stayed in one place, but the body twisted 180 degrees so that the brain, spinal cord, and spine together became dorsal to the gut.

At the risk of seeming obtuse, if the body twists relative to the head, yes, crossing of axons in a neuraxis would occur, but what about the esophagus: does it twist as well? Kinsbourne doesn't talk about the fate of the esophagus. Instead, he asks us to consider the location of the typical invertebrate heart. It lies dorsally, and blood gets pumped towards the belly, flows posteriorly, and returns to the heart dorsally. In a chordate or vertebrate, the heart is ventral, and blood pulsates to the dorsum, and returns to the heart via ventral, large veins. There's an invertebrate-to-vertebrate cardiovascular twist, it seems, to support Kinsbourne, but I still wonder about that esophagus. Does it untwist eventually in evolution for the survival of species, because all animals need to get food down somehow?

What matters most to Kinsbourne is the predictive power of his concept. He says that there should never be an organism–"no organism should come to light" are his precise words–in which the neuraxis is dorsal, but decussation is absent. He's clever, because he avoids saying that there can't be an organism with a ventral neuraxis in which decussation *does* occur. Worms with some decussating fibers aren't an impossibility.

The sample crossing that we mapped in drawing a pyramidal tract is a consequence of a momentous occurrence in evolution. The body didn't twist in relation to a fixed brain location in space specifically to create decussations. Fibers crossing the midline–or not crossing–could happen for myriad reasons, but if you buy the telos of a vertebrate body plan (with an endoskeletal spine, a dorsal neuraxis, dorsal brain, a ventral heart) then nerve fibers must cross. One could speak of a *sine qua non* of vertebrate existence: if vertebrate, then decussation perforce.

The student's question comes to mind once more: "OK, so why does the right brain have to do with left body and vice versa?" An answer, based on the first of our papers, would be: because crossing is an epiphenomenon. ("If you are a vertebrate . . . that's just the way it is" might be another way of saying the same thing.) The author talks about his model for the evolution of decussation, but the model isn't technically about decussation at all. It's about how vertebrates look anatomically in comparison to invertebrates. Indeed there are differences between the two types of living beings, but didn't we learn as much in some distant biology class?

3

Organization and Information

Next comes a perspective from engineering and mathematics. A virtue in this second of three papers is the attention it pays to sensory information directed to cortex. Consider the technical question the authors (bioengineer Shinbrot and neuroscientist Young, both mathematically inclined) pose: what are the constraints on getting information from one place to another? I'll take some liberty in explaining why constraints should enter into consideration at all. The following vignette is mine, not the authors', but it helps me begin to understand their paper and the concepts in it.

Let's say something lightly touches the dorsum of my left hand–in the middle of the dorsum of my left hand, just below the bottom of my middle finger, not as far down as the wrist. I know rather precisely where the touch is. In fact, I could touch the very spot in question with my right forefinger if asked to do so. How do I know that the touch didn't occur in the palm of my left hand? It's an absurd question, of course: the back of my left hand is where the information is, so to speak, not involving the palm at all.

When the touch happened, I neglected to mention that I had my left hand palm-side down, but not resting on anything. Now I flip my left hand palm-side up, and the touch happens again at exactly the same spot on the dorsum. The location of the touch in three-dimensional space has likely changed a bit. But the surface location of the stimulus on the left dorsum has not changed. A first constraint, almost too obvious to bother mentioning but important nonetheless, is that whatever pathways are involved in the perception of the light touch, the coordinates of location relate to my left hand, not some x, y, z location in extra-personal space.

We've described discrete events: 1. a touch on the dorsum of the left hand at a precise spot with the palm facing down and 2. a touch at the same spot on the dorsum with the palm facing up. If there were a map of some kind representing my hand, would there be one or two locations for the two events? If one answers "just one, on the dorsum" then how to account for the changed position of the left hand? The difference matters, because if I wanted to touch the spot on the left with my right forefinger, the task differs depending on whether my left hand is palm down or up. Does one need a different map, more three dimensional perhaps, in which the spot on the left dorsum gets two representations, one with the left hand palm-side down and another with the left hand palm-side up? Three dimensionality (any possible location of the hand in external space as the touch occurs) introduces not so much a constraint as a seemingly limitless quantity of information to be mapped somehow.

We spoke at the start about information getting from one place to another, so let's perform rudimentary connections between two maps. Map one–call it "actual left hand"–has a black dot on it, representing the spot of the touch, but for the sake of distinguishing dorsum from palm, we place a red dot on the flip side of Map one's surface (anywhere will do). Map two–call it "virtual left hand"–also has a black dot on it on its dorsum and likewise a red dot on the reverse, palmar side. Connect black dot with black dot and red with red (reading this chapter's paper had me playing with index cards and string; I literally did connect dots). Flip Map one 180 degrees, and there will be crossing of the strings, unless you flip Map two 180 degrees in the same direction.

The authors say that such point-to-point connectivity, when it comes to representing a three-dimensional location *on the virtual map*, is cumbersome. And it is without question, especially if you consider that connecting dots between actual and virtual maps would involve a surfeit of crossings if, for example, we tracked the progress of an ant walking across the dorsum of the hand towards the palm then down the side of a finger. Note that the crossing of strings between dots is not a decussation of fibers across the body's midline. In our vignette, the virtual map and the actual map are homolateral to each other. Pathways/strings between actual and virtual (by analogy, respectively: body map and hypothetical brain map) will crisscross, but no midline decussation occurs at all.

8

The authors think that an inescapable problem in representing three-dimensional sensory information is messiness and disorganization. Like a law that can't be violated without deleterious consequences, a constraint operates in the cortical representation of sensory data. It is a statute of neatness or efficiency. The telos is an unmessy, organized transfer of information from the periphery to the brain. In a modest edit of the medical student's question, how does decussation across a midline help to organize information, especially in three dimensions?

Now is a good time to review a pathway that has to do with the perception of light touch in humans, though it has been studied most carefully in other animals. Although we'll discuss the lemniscal system in particular, I'll direct attention to a structural feature that is also an aspect of another ascending tract mediating pain and temperature sensation.

The lightest touch on the dorsum, again, of the left hand is a phenomenon in and of itself that we could discuss for a while. Did hair follicles move with the touch? Did the touch involve some slight movement across the skin or just pressure in one place? Did the touch involve heat or cold? What is "touch"? To simplify, let's talk about a mechanical activation of some tactile corpuscles in the skin there, a bit of information that finds its way to consciousness, if we become aware that our left hand has been touched.

Light-touch sensory fibers in the peripheral nervous system are said to be generously myelinated with swift conduction times, but some investigators talk about a mix of degrees of myelination in sensory nerves mediating light touch. The cell bodies of the axons in question are located in a dorsal root ganglion, which lies in close proximity to the dorsal side of the spinal cord. (We'll concentrate on the left cervical cord, because the information comes from the dorsum of the left hand.) From the dorsal root ganglion, without a synapse, fibers will enter the cord heading into a fasciculus (a bundle) in the dorsal column of the cord. There's little argument about the amount of myelin in a dorsal column: the fascicles there are thickly myelinated.

We are now in the cuneate fasciculus–the column of Burdach, if you learn anatomy in Europe–in the dorsolateral left spinal cord. More specifically, there has been a transformation of mechanical activation into an electrical signal, and the signal (call it just one action potential, for the sake of simplicity) travels along myelinated axons in the cuneate fasciculus. A synapse will occur in the cuneate nucleus, located rostrally, at the cervicomedullary junction. I should call it by its proper name: it is the medial cuneate nucleus, because there's also a lateral (accessory) cuneate nucleus, which is associated with a different ascending tract to cerebellum rather than cerebrum.

Before the synapse in the medial cuneate nucleus occurs, where's the spot on the dorsum of the left hand represented?

We say that there is somatotopic organization at all levels of the lemniscal system, as is true for other somatic sensory pathways. Sensory information from the leg ascends in the dorsomedial cord in the gracile fasciculus, from the arm and hand dorsolaterally in the cuneate fasciculus; we refer to such parcellation as somatotopic. But a sense of anatomical order suggested by the word somatotopy needs to be adjusted when we think about how the hand is represented in the medial cuneate nucleus. In a portion of that nucleus called the *pars rotunda*, the hand's map is deconstructed and rearranged.

If, at this very moment, I look at the back of my left hand, I see, moving proximal to distal: my wrist, my dorsum, then my knuckled, wrinkled fingers. If I look at a coronal section of the *pars rotunda* in the medial cuneate nucleus, the representation of the hand, going dorsal to ventral, is: dorsum of hand, palm, dorsal fingertips, palmar fingertips—to simplify: back, front, back, front, with dorsum and palm *above* the fingers.

Maybe the above is knowledge that only an anatomist could love. The point is: before decussation across the midline (we'll trace it in a moment), there's a routing of connections to a curious-looking map of the hand in the medial cuneate nucleus. To create such a map likely necessitates crossings of connections just as in the flip of Map one relative to Map two that we described earlier.

Let's now track the course of the second-order neuron in the lemniscal system. As is also true in the anterolateral sensory pathway, a second-order neuron, not the first-order neuron, will cross the midline. From the medial cuneate nucleus, after a synapse, second-order axons cross from the left side to a medial, vertically oriented tract, the right medial lemniscus. The fibers arch through the central medulla on both sides (the internal arcuate fibers, which cross the midline). In the medial lemniscus, now in the right brainstem, representation of the left arm and hand is dorsal to that of the leg and foot. All the fibers, literally in a ribbon (a lemniscus), will wind their way rostrally towards the ventroposterior nuclear group of the right thalamus, then to right parietal cortex. The decussation of leminscal fibers happens a little higher (a bit more rostrally) than the decussation of the pyramidal tracts in the motor system.

The basic pathway that we have sketched invites mathematical considerations, according to our authors. The math involves the likelihood of wiring errors if the number of elements connected to each other is large and if the number of turns to be negotiated is also large. The authors say that a fully decussated arrangement across the midline of just 1,000 connections between brain and body maps, as opposed to an undecussated arrangement, reduces the probability of wiring error by at least an order of magnitude.

They offer a computer simulation (first using brain and body maps with 1,000 nodes each without decussation) to demonstrate that when you introduce a very small error factor each time over 100,000 iterations, then somatotopic correlation–the connections–between brain and body maps go very awry (and they stay that way) after just 10,000 trials. But in a decussated arrangement, rather few non-somatotopic connections ever arise at any point in the simulation, well past the 10,000 mark by an order of magnitude. Since miswiring in neurobiology is inherently disadvantageous and because error in complex systems is inescapable, there "should be an evolutionary drive toward decussated networks," because the best way to transfer information is to keep it organized and as error free as possible.

I'll draw an analogy to a hypothetical city divided by a river that runs east to west. I'm interested to get from point A in the southwest of the city to point B northeast. My plan is to take a subway, and my station can be found at the center of the city on the northern bank of the river. Crossing at that one place reduces the possibility of my getting lost in getting from south to north or, for that matter, north to south.

Fibers decussate after synapsing in the medial caudate nucleus. In that nucleus, the map of the hand already looks different than my left hand, and we know very well that the homuncular representations in thalamus and sensory cortex exaggerate–they even reduplicate–some parts of the body while maintaining a semblance of somatotopy.

We simply can't talk about a single homuncular representation anywhere in the subsequent course of the lemniscal pathway after its decussation. Sensory cortical maps, taking just Brodmann's areas 3a (at the bottom of the central sulcus), 3b (caudal bank of central sulcus), 1 (a large part of the postcentral gyrus, visible on the lateral surface), and 2 (caudal to 1, but without extension to the medial surface of the brain), reduplicate homuncular representations. The multiple homunculi lie in a columnar arrangement next to each other in Brodmann's areas 3a, 3b, 1, and 2.

Then there's the anterolateral system, which we've not traced in detail, except to notice that second-order neurons also cross the midline in that distinct ascending system. Second-order fibers arise after synapsing in the *substantia gelatinosa* to cross segmentally in the cord in anterior white commissures at many levels. After crossing, the anterolateral system ascends on the opposite side towards the thalamus and cortex. The parsimony afforded by decussation, i.e., a reduced error rate, might still apply if we think about the pathway mediating pain and temperature, but why so many crossings?

The interest in Shinbrot and Young's paper is its claim that decussation is anything but a random biological phenomenon. It occurred for the limitation of wrong connections. It's a lovely argument, but the anatomy is even more beautiful and humbling than the authors' mathematics.

4

The Singular Phenomenon
of Decussation

The title of this chapter is a phrase of Cajal's. The third of our papers owes much to his cogitation on the incomplete crossing of fibers in the visual system—which we will discuss in what follows. But, in their first pages, the authors (Vulliemoz, Raineteau, and Jabaudon) teach me a fact which I'll accept at face value; it's worth a moment's consideration: in non-mammalian vertebrates, tracts that originate in the brainstem control *most* motor functions. By "most," they refer to practicalities such as control of muscular tone, of posture, and the maintenance of balance of an entire body. Tracts arising in the brainstem are numerous, but a short list would include: reticulospinal, tectospinal, vestibulospinal, and rubrospinal. Which of these cross the midline?

Let me phrase the question differently. Would you expect all of them *not* to cross the midline? We have introduced the lateral vestibulospinal tract arising from Deiters' lateral vestibular nucleus, and we said that it facilitates extensor tone on the same side of the body without decussation across the midline. It would make teaching and memorization so much easier if we could say, "if a descending motor tract arises in the brainstem, then it's an uncrossed tract." The statement isn't true, unfortunately, but I find it interesting that, depending on where a brainstem motor tract originates, some cross the midline and others don't.

Officially to answer the question, then, the tectospinal and rubrospinal tracts (arising from the superior colliculus and red nucleus, respectively) cross the midline, whereas the reticulospinal and vestibulospinal tracts (arising from pontine and medullary portions of the reticular formation and medullary vestibular nuclei, respectively) do not. Someone will object that reticulospinal fibers sometimes do cross the midline at a lower point, maybe in the low medulla or in the spinal cord. That person, even if technically correct, misses the singularity that Cajal observes about decussations.

They are singularly obvious. It doesn't take effort to see the decussation of the pyramids at the cervicomedullary junction: it effaces the anterior median fissure on the ventral surface. Intraaxially, we can see decussating internal arcuate fibers in the transition from the medial caudate or gracile nuclei to the medial lemnisci on either side. Likewise, tectospinal tracts manifestly cross in a dorsal tegmental decussation in midbrain. And rubrospinal tracts cross in a ventral tegmental decussation in the midbrain. At the level of the third nerve nuclear complex (visualize a canonical axial microphotograph of a midbrain, with obvious red nuclei and the shark tooth appearance of nucleus of cranial nerve III in the middle), a lot of midline crossing happens near and around those red nuclei. Consider, as an additional example, the decussation of the superior cerebellar peduncles just caudal to the level just mentioned. Decussation simply isn't subtle; it's a plain phenomenon. Crossings across the midline vexed Cajal, because their functional benefit to an organism struck him as "obscure" (his word).

So, in non-mammalian vertebrates, brainstem pathways control most motor functions. What's to be done after most control has been achieved? The authors talk about exceptional motor capacities that supervene once most motor control has been accomplished. As the telencephalon develops in size and complexity from non-mammal to the human mammal, is decussation necessary for increasingly exceptional capacities? The authors say yes.

*

Let's consider a particularly obvious chiasm in anatomy.

About 165 years before Cajal, Isaac Newton anatomized binocular vision. Here is query 15 from Book Three of his *Opticks* (note that this third part of the book is a series of questions, rather than the "propositions" one finds elsewhere in the work): "Are not the Species of Objects seen with both Eyes united where the optick Nerves meet before they come into the

Brain, the Fibres on the right side of both Nerves uniting there, and after union going thence into the Brain in the Nerve [what we would now call the tract] which is on the right side of the Head . . . [?] . . . For the optick Nerves of such Animals as look the same way with both Eyes (as of Men, Dogs, Sheep, Oxen, &c) meet before they come into the Brain, but the optick Nerves of such Animals as do not look the same way with both Eyes (as of Fishes, and of the Chameleon) do not meet, if I am rightly inform'd."

In response to Sir Isaac, who is neuroanatomically correct about the human optic chiasm, I'll digress briefly.

Since my own introductory anatomy days in school, I've wondered whether animals who have eyes on the sides of their heads, who seem to look laterally rather than in a forward direction, have optic chiasms or visual pathway decussations. Then, one day–in one of those scholarly fishing expeditions that can occupy a person for a whole afternoon or more–I found a paper entitled "Stereopsis in Toads." Like chameleons, toads have quite laterally displaced eyes, but unlike chameleons, to make matters apparently worse for toads, toads' eyes barely move in their sockets. Yet toads achieve depth perception (stereopsis); they have optic chiasms; and–here's a remarkable observation–toads have a visual field of almost 360 degrees, due to binocular overlap that is both in front of and, importantly, *above* the eyes. I'll spare the reader comments about the visually-guided accuracy of a toad's tongue dart for food in three-dimensional space. The take-home from my digression is, simply, that "Animals as do not look the same way with both Eyes" nevertheless have chiasms. Newton was slightly misinformed.

Vulliemoz, Raineteau, and Jabaudon invoke Cajal's conjecture (from 1898) that, in the course of evolution, the more fibers cross in an optic chiasm the *less* likely one would observe decussating motor fibers. Does the inverse relationship make sense? A visual datum in left external space transmits to the right brain of a vertebrate without limbs. Let's say that the crossing is absolutely complete: all ganglion cell axons from the left retina transmit to the right brain. Then (so runs the conjecture) descending, uncrossed motor pathways in the right brain drive movement in the right hemibody–for example, the right side contracts to evade or extends to approach the datum in left external space. There's no need for a decussating motor pathway.

To consider a more exceptional task under visual guidance, we need to know about a visual pathway that doesn't completely cross.

I'll start with ganglion cells in the retina, because we 're discussing a fiber tract. The outgoing axons in question belong to retinal ganglion cells. Not all ganglion cells connect to other retinal cells the same way. At the fovea (or macula), one cone connects to one bipolar cell then to one retinal ganglion cell. Elsewhere, the connection is less one to one. For the retina as a whole, the ratio of all light receptors (cones and rods) to ganglion cells is estimated to be 125:1.

In the periphery of the retina, as opposed to the fovea, more cones and rods connect to more bipolar cells, which connect to the relatively parsimonious number of ganglion cells. The fovea, just to state what's well known, is responsible for our acutest vision. And in the fovea, retinal ganglion axons in its nasal half are destined to cross the midline, those in the temporal half will not. The naso-temporal division is not always clear in other species, but in primates and humans, it's very sharp.

Temporal retinal and foveal fibers that don't cross terminate in various locations, among them the pretectal nuclei, the superior colliculus, and even the suprachiasmatic nucleus in hypothalamus, in addition to the lateral geniculate nucleus, all on the same side. Fibers that do cross—only those nasal to the nasotemporal division of the whole retina and its fovea—will terminate in the contralateral superior colliculus and lateral geniculate nucleus, not to the other locations just mentioned.

Whether crossing in the visual pathway is complete or partial, our authors tell us, depends on the existence of binocular vision—or, stereopsis. In brief, they offer us two claims to consider. First, partial crossing is necessary for stereopsis. Second, stereopsis is so necessary for exceptional motor acts that the pathways responsible for those acts (like the corticospinal tract) will decussate in relationship to the development of stereopsis. Though I don't doubt that binocular vision is a useful attribute for tasks performed under visual guidance, I have a problem with the second claim, based on the anatomy that supports the first. I also hear the medical student quizzing me with exasperation: "The corticospinal tract crosses, because the visual pathway partially crosses, because we're visual animals? Really?"

The lateral geniculate nucleus (also known as the lateral geniculate body) is the terminus of the optic tract. One of my teachers had this to say about binocular vision and that nucleus (from a book entitled *Eye, Brain, and Vision*): "The lateral geniculate body represents the first opportunity for information from the two eyes to come together at the level of a single cell. But it seems that the opportunity there is missed: the two sets of input are consigned to separate sets of layers, with little or no opportunity to combine. As we would expect from this segregation, a geniculate cell responds to one eye and not at all to the other."

The opportunity is missed rather completely, in fact. Among the six cellular layers of the lateral geniculate nucleus, any one layer or any cell in that one layer deals either with left or right eye information, despite the fact that fibers from both eyes converge in the lateral geniculate nucleus. For stereopsis to happen, information kept so very discrete must merge somewhere. Question: where? My teacher's answer is: the cerebral cortex and at no point prior to it. The comment stuns by its simplicity.

I have a task in mind as I describe the visual pathway and its relationship to motor control. I'm threading a needle. Certainly it's a task under visual guidance. The high likelihood is that I perform this act in a well-lit place, and odds are that the needle and thread are oriented toward my foveae. I want to maximize the likelihood of success on my first attempt. I've already moistened the thread, which I hold between my right thumb and forefinger; the eye of the needle faces my eyes, which point inwardly in slight accommodation. The needle in fixed in space, more or less (due to my little tremor), with my left forefinger and thumb. Like some often do, I close one eye, because it seems I see better with one eye than the other. In my case, I close my left eye just for a moment. I thread the needle. Was stereopsis involved?

At least both motor cortices—whatever controls movement in both my hands—must be engaged in this task, which requires that I know where objects are in space and at what relative depth. One surmises that stereopsis must be involved, with activity in visual cortex.

All of a sudden, questions come to mind. Which visual cortex? Cortex on both sides? When I close my left eye to spot the eye of the needle keenly, don't I temporarily yield binocularity? But monocular information from my right eye reaches both cortices—nasal right retinal information heads to left cortex by crossing the midline; temporal right retinal information heads to right cortex without crossing. We've traced the pathway as far as the lateral geniculate nucleus, which only has cells specific to right or left eye. Truly binocular cells are a cortical matter, as my teacher said. For a fine motor skill, performed just in front of my midline (in front of my nose, actually), I'd say that a whole lot of my cortex—motoric and visual—is active, on both sides. Stereopsis simply invites consideration of how both cortices can be involved in trivial needle threading.

I can't wholly agree with the authors when they suggest that visual wiring influenced the development of a decussating corticospinal tract. They rephrase Cajal's conjecture, and of course it's an affront to disagree with a Cajal. But what does "influence" mean? It's a squishy verb.

We can say instead that there must be a lot of midline crossing in motor and visual systems alike for information to get where it needs to go in the task of needle threading. Both cerebral cortices are likely involved, and the hemispheres must engage each other—they must communicate in real time—somehow.

*

The remainder of the third paper in our series has to do with syndromes in which decussations are absent, with a variety of clinical consequences. One of the syndromes, first described in the late 1960's, will be a topic later. For now, we're not done discussing a basic anatomy of crossings, but we're in a position to summarize what all three papers have taught us so far.

One doubts that the fabled missing link will be found, the first or ur-vertebrate whose body twists up to 180 degrees relative to the brain. Vertebrate and chordate body plans inescapably have dorsal neuraxes and endoskeletons, but it's a misstatement to say that crossing doesn't happen in invertebrates. In a vertebrate, however, crossing results in a bicameral arrangement in which one half of the brain represents or deals with the opposite half of space.

Depicting space in three dimensions on a cortical map—the main subject matter of the second paper of the three I chose—is a non-trivial information problem prone to error, and maybe midline decussation organizes data.

A question as benign as "forget decussations for a moment, why are there even *tracts* in anatomy?" begins to resemble the medical student's original question in kind. Why tracts at all? A tract keeps like fibers together in discrete boulevards; similarly, decussation allows like fibers to achieve their analogous positions on cortical maps with less likelihood of losing their way. The answer to queries about tracts and decussations is: less error, to which biology and life is prone.

Then, based on a conjecture by Cajal, the authors of the third paper contemplate actions performed by the nervous system when most motor control has been achieved. We've considered a task requiring bimanual dexterity performed right in front of eyes pointing forward, and we infer that halves of the brain are communicating to accomplish the threading of a needle.

Crossing is manifest in brain anatomy. A non-mundane question arises because of that singular phenomenon. It's a question in two parts. We basically discuss sidedness—right side of brain, left side of the world, etc. When do sides happen in the brain? Then: how do sides communicate?

We need more anatomy, because we haven't at all exhausted how much crossing there is.

5

Start from Scratch

If there's one course in medical school, or part of a course, that I'd take again from scratch, it would be embryology. Dusting off my copy of Langman's *Medical Embryology*, which was in its fourth edition in the 1980's, I turn to the last chapter, on the central nervous system. (It seems that the nervous system occupies the backside of all general medical textbooks.) Way back when, by the time I got to Langman's chapter 20, the embryology final exam was imminent, my exhaustion complete, and the intellect dissipated. But it's the neuro-development part of the course I'd retake today. I read on the chapter's first page that a flattish thickening of ectoderm, called a neural plate, appears early in the third gestational week in humans, and that closure of the cranial neuropore occurs around day 25.

Fast forward from a horrid first year of school to the second year of neurology training, during months at a place then abbreviated TCH, for *The* Children's Hospital, as opposed to a children's hospital. There, a teacher of sphinx-like demeanor taught that a given brain malformation may not have its onset after a developmental event is completed. The statement–in fact, it was an end-stop pronouncement that left silence in its wake–strikes me as a riddle to this day. Here's a variation of the riddle for present purposes: when do right and left connect in brains? We ask, not only because we want to know when connections start, but also when they might go astray.

Upon closure of the cranial neuropore, in what is otherwise called induction on the dorsal side of the embryo (there's yet another synonym:

---

dorsal induction is also known as primary neurulation), is *that* when right and left connect?

Take out another index card (this time it's my model of a neural plate). Indulge me by drawing a thick line with a Sharpie right down the middle of the card lengthwise. We'll call this line the ventral extent of tube. Appose the left and right side of the card, with the Sharpie line on the inside of the tube. Apply tape to the seam along the whole length. The tape marks the dorsal side.

I've joined right and left sides of the card together, but the only demarcations are the Sharpie line and the dorsal seam. We have modeled dorsal induction.

To make my index-card exercise a bit more rigorous, I head to a website like Online Mendelian Inheritance in Man. I enter "dorsal neural tube induction." Like a jackpot on the computer screen, there's immediately more genetics in front of me than I can know at a glance. There are names like wingless, snail family transcriptional repressor (slug), bone morphogenetic protein (BMP), paired box (PAX), sonic hedgehog (SHH), many more. In the aggregate, the talk is about dorsal vs. ventral genetic expression, not right vs. left. For example, wingless proteins (Wnt) are found more on the dorsal side of the neural tube; sonic hedgehog (the protein) concentrates ventrally. The molecular mechanisms of induction are the stuff of current embryology courses, as students today know all too well.

The great sphinx of TCH would say that once dorsal induction and closure of the cranial neuropore occurs, you can't *not* have a brain, as in cases of craniorachischisis totalis or anencephaly. Unanswered, however, is the matter of right and left sides and the connections between the two. The cranial neuropore was once an open end to the neural tube; it closes by apposition of its sides as guided by multiple genes and their proteins. Do interhemispheric connections happen at that time? The Sphinx shrugs in response. "At this time, there are no hemispheres," I hear him in my ear.

Dorsal induction happens at approximately three to four weeks' gestation. Ventral induction happens at approximately five-to-six weeks' gestation. To get as efficiently as possible to our interest at five-to-six weeks, look back a few sentences to note the word "ventral" (as in ventral neural tube) associated with sonic hedgehog, the protein. Its gene, SHH, is located on chromosome seven; its expression happens along the ventral neural tube in the midline.

Now, consider three observations together: 1. Ventral induction, when complete after the sixth week, results in *paired* cerebral hemispheres; the *corpus callosum* across hemispheres myelinates (appears) later; 2. There can't be onset of holoprosencephaly after the fifth or sixth week, but when it occurs, the most severe cases are characterized by an undivided cortical mantle, a midline single ventricle, no olfactory bulbs or tracts, sometimes a single optic nerve to a cyclopean eye, typically no *corpus callosum*, and cortical histology that looks like hippocampal archicortex; 3. A spectrum of SHH mutations causes holoprosencephaly with diverse phenotypes, not all of them affecting the brain to the severest extent just mentioned.

After five-to-six weeks' gestation and after successful ventral induction, then and only then can one discuss hemispheric division under the influence of SHH (that gene, at very least). And there can't yet be any meaningful mention of neuronal connections, because myelination of axons will occur in a sequence that extends in time well past the sixth week even into young adulthood.

Actually, a first observation about connectivity in the early fetal brain might be that there's no myelin–so, essentially, no connections. Instead, we have a TCH mantra pertinent to the first month and a half of existence. CLOSE, first (closure of the cranial neuropore); DIVIDE, second (into cerebral hemispheres); PROLIFERATE, last (neurons begin to proliferate and to migrate no earlier than at eight weeks' gestation). There's a hint of irony in all the above: you've divided left from right with no connection between what you've divided; in the first weeks of gestation, wiring isn't hard-wired.

By the way, when ventral induction occurs, the rudimentary brain doesn't only divide along the long axis. There's division in all axes: x, y, and z. Dividing top from bottom in a simplified brain sphere, we can visualize a basal (ventral/motor) versus an alar (dorsal/sensory) hemisphere. The demarcation (call it the x axis) is the *sulcus limitans* of Wilhelm His, Senior (his son, also an academic physician, described the heart's bundle of His); the *sulcus limitans* is particularly obvious in the spinal cord and the medulla oblongata. The y axis is the horizontal midline. On either side of the y axis, just now beginning to expand into z-axis space, we have the nascent hemispheres.

Paired, lateral hemispheres are the interest here. There's an ontogeny of connections between the two sides which we can review, mainly to note how much of a work-in-progress it is getting hemispheres to wire. The decussating tracts mentioned in our earlier chapters are only a small part of the crossed organization of brains.

*

Like an editor fussy about diction, the medical student groans at the word *ontogeny* and begrudgingly looks up a definition, "the course of development of an individual organism." Given that a different book could be written about what we now know about fetal and post-birth human myelination, a brief ontogenic review can only highlight moments in a sequence that most of us have negotiated successfully. We're interested to describe when midline connections happen and where they happen, in embryologic time.

Back to our index card. As we left it, we just had a tube with a ventral Sharpie line and a dorsal seam, nothing more. To visualize ventral induction in the fifth-to-sixth week, pinch the tube on its cranial end, then look down the tube's long axis. Look towards the rostral pinch. (If you insist, you can try push up just from the ventral side, in deference to ventral induction, but just pinching one end–top and bottom together–works.)

Use your imagination, and think that you are looking through a midline ventricle (in my mind, I think the third ventricle) into the start of two lateral ventricles. The ventral Sharpie line and the dorsal seam meet in the middle where you are pinching. In this crude model, where the lines converge–at the pinch–marks the lamina terminalis in anatomy, the rostral extent of the third ventricle.

I stare down the length of the dorsal seam. My Sharpie line looks like it returns back to me ventrally, towards the center of my gaze. We can map the locations of crossings which first appear in the tenth gestational week, though, at week ten, many appear as mere shadows or premonitions compared to their mature forms.

A caveat: in terms of an axial level, we'll begin at the start of the third ventricle, so we won't comment on two interesting, more caudal crossings, the trochlear decussation and the medial longitudinal fasciculus. Those are topics for the next chapter.

The following six names may not all be familiar; I'll help with crib notes next to the names. Each of them cross the midline. Beginning dorsally, they are:

1. The posterior commissure (Think about the pupillary light reflex: how does light presented to one pupil get transferred, as information, to the other side?).
2. The habenular commissure. (From my Latin dictionary: habenula, diminutive of habena, "that by which a thing is held," like a horse rider's rein or a strap. The habenula and the pineal gland are very close to each other: how does light influence sleep?)
3. We move more ventrally:
4. *Corpus callosum*, literally hard body, is anterior to the lamina terminalis. It's utterly rudimentary, hardly hard, at ten weeks.
5. The hippocampal or fornical commissure, which may appear a bit later than ten weeks (fourteen weeks, according to anatomist Nieuwenhuys et al., 2008).
6. The anterior commissure. I'll comment on it in a moment.
7. The optic chiasm, whose myelination continues well into the seventh gestational month.

Of these six, the anterior commissure, which connects olfactory areas of the nascent cortices and the amygdalae on either side, is the first to appear. Next come the habenular and posterior commissures. The oldest tissues connect first (think: olfactory areas, habenulae, hippocampal formations). The new cortices (think: via *corpus callosum*) connect later.

Enlisting the hint about a posterior commissure connecting side to side in a visual pathway that has to do with external space, do these six commissures interconnect a divided brain, body, and map of the external world? There are two ways to answer. First, a too-simplistic response: yes, because sides meet. Alternatively, we might obsess over the word commissure (literally, a commitment–which is different than an accomplished connection.

Based on anatomy in the midline third ventricle at ten weeks' gestation, phylogenetically old brain starts to connect to with old brain on the other side, like aged alumnae/alumni who reconnect at a dreary reunion. Someone will complain that I haven't defined old versus new brain anatomically, and that's quite correct, perhaps unforgivable. But if you want an example of a really old strap of neural tissue, the habenula is an archetype, a better example than even amygdala or hippocampus. The habenular commissure connects very old side its kindred on the other side.

*

The clock of life now reads ten weeks' gestation. Notice at this moment, there's no representation of the body, really. We have no medial lemniscus, no internal capsule, no pyramidal tract, no decussation of pyramids, and not even much of an optic chiasm.

So, when do right body and left brain and vice versa enter into their fixed and irreversible commitment to each other?

6

An Aside on Eyes Moving Conjugately

Some poor soul, a mature adult, suffers an infarction in the right hemisphere. The left body is weak, arm weaker than leg. The eyes look together, conjugately, to the right; the head turns to the right as well.

Looking away from hemiparesis (towards the lesion) in a case of cortical infarction was the subject of a 19th-century thesis by a Genevan named Jean-Louis Prévost, based on his clinical experience in Paris. He reported 51 cases. His Parisian mentor, Alfred Vulpian, gave him the idea to study the phenomenon.

Depending on the size and location of the responsible lesion in the hemisphere, deviation of the eyes can last days to weeks, but it isn't permanent. Acutely, if well enough to follow instructions, the patient would be able to look up and down when asked to do so, with both eyes moving together. But the eyes still deviate conjugately to the right in the horizontal plane.

This chapter addresses two issues having to do with eyes.

Here's the first of the two: why do eye abduction and contralateral eye adduction (and vice versa) happen together in the first place? Many medical students can't wait to blurt out the words "medial longitudinal fasciculus" (or the letters M, L, and F). Not to be harsh, but that's not an answer. The medial longitudinal fasciculus (MLF) is just a name.

It's true that the MLF contains a decussating connection between an abducens nucleus on one side and that part of the oculomotor nucleus that controls the medial rectus on the opposite side. (One adds quickly that the MLF contains much else. In fact, the majority of its fibers originate in vestibular nuclei, *not* the abducens nucleus.) It's also true that in the absence of an MLF, or if it were damaged in some way, the conjugate deviation we've described in the case of a right hemisphere stroke might differ. The MLF pertains to our discussion, absolutely.

But to answer the first of our two questions, we're on firmer ground with a less sophisticated answer, which smacks of teleology (not always good), but it is simple and not simplistic (usually good): Assuming we aren't blind in one eye, for us to be able to move our eyes in the horizontal plane, one eye has to abduct *as* the other adducts. For good measure, we can mention equal innervation of abductor and adductor, because without it (per Ewald Hering's law of equal innervation), we run the chance of double vision with any horizontal saccade. Of note, we're not just talking about voluntary saccades towards objects in the periphery.

If my head subtly moves from side to side, to keep an object in front of me on my retinae (foveae), the eyes must move conjugately in the horizontal plane, in a direction opposite to the head movement. Prévost's observation that the head as well as the eyes turn to the side of the lesion (he says so in the title of his thesis, *De la déviation conjugée des yeux et de la rotation de la tete dans certain cas d'hemiplegie*) becomes a nuance of interest. Eyes (*des yeux*) rivet to the right; the patient literally rotates the head/*la tete* in that same direction, as if willfully gazing away from her or his paralysis. But it's not a willed act.

I should make an important distinction regarding gaze. There are countless gazes, as artists know (Picasso acknowledged a native Andalusian *mirada fuerte*–strong gazing–as a birthright important to his art).

A neurologist distinguishes between a visually evoked movement of eyes with long latency, on the order of 100 milliseconds, and very short latency eye movements which transpire more quickly by a factor of ten, or roughly 10 milliseconds. Short latency is necessary to make the kinds of vertical, torsional, and horizontal compensations required when the head subtly moves in all planes when walking, running, etc. Short-latency eye movements have to do with the vestibulo-ocular reflex, a neural matrix of brainstem connections. Long-latency gaze, including Andalusian strong gazing, involves more of the entire brain.

We ended our last chapter curious about timing, when one side of brain definitively links to the other side of the body. In the case of the MLF, we're awfully close to definitiveness: two nuclei on opposite sides connect to each other; midline crossing happens (must happen); and the structure myelinates early.

Anatomist Brodal (1981) says the MLF is phylogenetically ancient, and "in ontogenesis it stands out very clearly on account of its early myelination." We've discussed commissures whose primordial forms can be seen at 10 weeks' gestation. The MLF appears even earlier, at the end of the first gestational month. In many vertebrates, the MLF is the very first white-matter tract to appear in ontogeny. At full-term birth in humans, there's a short list of structures whose myelination is visible in a gross dissection. On that list are: MLF, cranial nerves, the optic chiasm and tracts (but not the optic radiations), and some other structures whose myelination is not quite as clear as the others.

*

With respect to vertical conjugate movements of eyes, here is the second of two issues in this chapter, phrased again as a question: why do eye elevation and contralateral eye extorsion happen together in the first place? I hear the medical student in a state of consternation: "what in the world *is* 'extorsion,' as opposed to the criminal act of extortion?" Issue two in this chapter is completely analogous to issue one, but we refer now to vertical rather than horizontal movement.

The general subject is why individual ocular muscles are yoked in the first place. Assuming we aren't blind in one eye, for us to be able to move our eyes in the vertical plane, one eye has to elevate *as* the other extorts. For good measure, we can mention equal innervation of muscles which elevate and extort, because without it (per Ewald Hering's law of equal innervation), we run the chance of double vision with any vertical saccade. Decussation is involved in the yoking of muscles; indeed, decussation has to be involved.

Regarding extorsion as opposed to extortion as opposed to elevation, look up and to your left. Your right eye extorts as your left eye elevates. Now look down and to your right. Your right eye depresses as your left eye intorts.

We've mentioned short and long latencies in generating conjugate eye movements. In the case of quick vertical compensations, we should think about a rostral part of the MLF, high up in the midbrain, at the level of the upper pole of the red nucleus. Dorsal to the red nuclei at their very tips are nuclei of the rostral interstitial MLF.

Let's orient ourselves in the midbrain for a moment. Superior colliculus is above the inferior colliculus, check. Third nerve nucleus, including its various subnuclei, is above the trochlear nucleus, the latter roughly at the level of the inferior colliculus, check. The nuclei of the rostral interstitial MLF sits just above the upper pole of the red nucleus in the high midbrain. OK, you kindly say, I'll take your word for it.

Wait, there are subnuclei of the third nerve nucleus? Yes. There are subnuclei specific to the extraocular muscles controlled by the third cranial nerve. Those muscles are the inferior oblique, the inferior rectus, the superior rectus, and the medial rectus. In terms of vertical movement of eyes, there's something unique about fibers emanating from the subnucleus associated with the superior rectus. There's also something unique about the fibers emanating from the cranial nerve nucleus of the trochlear nerve, the fourth cranial nerve. What's the uniqueness?

The word "decussation" comes to mind.

They say, whoever they are, that only one cranial nerve has its nucleus on the side opposite where the muscle it innervates (textbook answer: a left trochlear nucleus gives rise to the right trochlear nerve, which innervates the right superior oblique). The trochlear midline crossing happens in the anterior medullary velum, which is a veil of tissue that stretches between the two superior cerebellar peduncles on the dorsal side of midbrain. Likewise, right trochlear nucleus innervates left superior oblique. The trochlear decussation is present at ten weeks' gestation in humans.

The trochlear nucleus has a partner in decussation. What we generically teach about the curiosity of the fourth cranial nerve sniffs of misstatement.

Fibers of the superior rectus subnucleus of cranial nerve III *also cross the midline*. The left subnucleus of cranial nerve III gives rise to fibers that innervate the right superior rectus muscle.

There's an elegance in the above informational overload. There's no other word for it: elegance.

Consider that a quick vertical (upward) corrective saccade is necessary, because in a run we take one random day, with one footfall, there's a pothole we didn't expect. It's an irregular pothole. A foot gets caught in an oblique way, casting us in an oblique downward direction, but, mercifully, we don't fall. The run continues to our satisfaction, without injury.

As foot meets pothole, I envision events having occurred within just a few milliseconds: unilateral firing of the rostral interstitial nucleus of the MLF, say, on the left, then immediate activation of the following, all on the same side of the midline (on the left): subnuclei of inferior oblique, inferior rectus, superior rectus, *and* the left trochlear nucleus. The result, with short latency between nuclear discharge and muscle action involving the eyes: a corrective saccade involving the left inferior oblique and inferior rectus acting on the left eye, and an equal saccade of contralateral superior rectus and the superior oblique acting on the right eye.

An irksomely assiduous student now wants to know about gaze with longer latency. She or he asks insistently, peering at me with Andalusian *mirada fuerte*. I tell that student that the interstitial nucleus of Cajal is involved in *mirada fuerte* (probably not the rostral interstitial nucleus of the MLF), but, not to worry: what we should do right now is relax, stop, think. What we've reviewed is sufficient for our purpose. You have to control *both* eyes, right? And you have to do so adhering all the while to Ewald Hering's law of equal innervation involving eyes on either side of the midline.

Yoked muscles necessitate decussation. The MLF and the trochlear decussation are eminently apparent at gestational week ten.

7

After the Tenth Week

I have a friend and colleague who tried once, on a stratospherically ambitious whim, to teach neuroanatomy to twelve students . . . just using words. No photomicrographs, no Powerpoint presentations, not even the dissection of brains. His course occupied a two-month block in the curriculum, back in the days when true experiments in pedagogy were encouraged at my medical school. I'm all for that freedom and always will be, but, at the time, I thought he was nuts. He said that the exercise tasked him—and, more importantly, forced his students—to communicate what's important as lucidly as possible. I'll adopt his odd but brilliant approach.

Chapter before last, we left off at the tenth week of gestation. Commissures and decussations are just visible. In the lower brainstem, we have the medial longitudinal fasciculus and the trochlear decussation.

Above and below the third ventricle, we have dorsal and ventral crossings. The posterior commissure is dorsal. The anterior commissure and the primordial *corpus callosum* are anterior and more ventral. The optic chiasm is most ventral. According to a mantra of brain development, we have CLOSED the cranial neuropore and DIVIDED into rudimentary cerebral hemispheres. Lower down, in the brainstem, we've also DIVIDED orthogonally to the long-axial midline into a basal (ventral) plate versus an alar (dorsal) plate; the demarcation between the two is the *sulcus limitans* of His.

Beginning no earlier than the eighth week, neurons PROLIFERATE. They do so well past the tenth week. Where do the neurons proliferate and where do they go?

*

In the midbrain at 5-10 gestational weeks, there's a tectum and a tegmentum that roughly correlate to the alar and basal plates, respectively. In the diencephalon at 5-10 weeks, we no longer have a basal plate at all; we only have an alar plate.

The diencephalon and structures rostral to it are *all* of alar origin. The diencephalic ventral alar plate will have (more or less) only motor nuclei, just as the basal plate is motoric in the brainstem and spinal cord. The diencephalic dorsal alar plate will have (more or less) only sensory nuclei, just as the alar plate is sensory in the brainstem and spinal cord.

In this developing diencephalon, the ventral alar part matures into hypothalamus, the dorsal alar part into thalamus (and more, as we'll see).

To conceptualize where neuroblasts, fated to become cortical neurons, proliferate, think about a most bizarre open-faced sandwich. It's a hollow sphere of bread covered by whatever you like on your bread—say, it's peanut butter. The hollow of the sphere is the third ventricle. The lower half of the spherical sandwich is ventral alar, destined to be hypothalamus; the upper half is dorsal alar, destined to be thalamus as well as cortex. Viewed from the outside, we see no bread in our structure. It looks like a sphere of peanut butter.

Now we apply anatomical terms to our sandwich. Bread equals a so-called mantle layer.[1] Peanut butter equals a so-called marginal layer. Early neurons pseudostratify in the mantle layer. The marginal layer contains pluripotent neuroepithelial cells, some of which will differentiate into glial cells.

Cells that mature into cortical neurons proliferate in the bread on the inside, not the peanut butter on the outside.

The hemispheres derive entirely from the dorsal half of our sandwich, *only* from the dorsal alar plate. Neocortical neurons originate in the dorsal

---

[1]   "Mantle layer" in my analogy conflates so-called matrix and mantle layers. And I do not mention the innermost ependymal layer, again for the sake of simplicity.

mantle layer, but they migrate across the dorsal marginal layer to form bread on the outside.

The dorsal half of our open-faced sandwich, with peanut butter on the outside, metamorphoses into a proper sandwich consisting of two pieces of bread and peanut butter between the slices. Outside bread equals developing neocortex. Peanut butter equals white matter deep to neocortex. Inside bread equals the mantle layer.

The two-piece-of-bread sandwich is temporary. To steal a peek at the telos or endpoint, we'll eventually re-achieve an open-faced sandwich with bread on the outside and peanut butter on the inside.

*

The life clock now reads three months' gestation.

We have before us a curious, bilobed sandwich.

Radial migration across the dorsal marginal layer forms bread on the outside. Neuronal proliferation and radial migration are robust, so much so that the outer bread layer eventually folds upon itself in literal gyrations. The two hemispheres connect to each other by a growing *corpus callosum*, which had started as a primordium just anterior to the anterior commissure. By the fifteen week of gestation, the *corpus callosum* forms a roof over the third ventricle. More and more white-matter axons cross the midline to the other hemisphere.

Neurons travel radially to get from the mantle layer across the marginal layer to the surface, but not all deep-bread neurons migrate in that way. Grey matter structures like the thalamus, *corpus striatum*, claustrum, amygdala, and olfactory cortex take their origin in the dorsal mantle layer and their neurons remain deep to the dorsal marginal layer.

The dorsal mantle layer dissipates in time.

The neocortex (bread on the outside) forms up to six layers of neurons; the underlying peanut-butter layer thickens as white matter becomes increasingly abundant.

Another great task is underway as the second trimester proceeds, aside from development of neocortex just described. Tracts form. They differ from interhemispheric commissures in that they cross from one side of the body towards the brain on the contralateral side, not from one side of the brain to the other. These ascending, decussating sensory pathways appear before the first hints of a descending corticospinal tract in ontogeny.

8

Fate

When we read about an axonal fate either to cross or not to cross the midline, there's a tendency to refer to axons as if they possessed intelligence and indulged fastidious, personal preferences. For example, an axon *recognizes* the axial midline; it is *attracted* to it or *repelled* by it; if it crosses the midline, it does so like Caesar crossing his river Rubicon, fated never to return. My etymological dictionary tells me that axon has its root in the word axis. Axons and axes relate to each other. I'm interested to understand some basics about axons and the body's midline, since commissures and decussations both traverse it. There's a great deal of literature that we might review. As has been obvious from the start, however, my goal hasn't been an encyclopedic review of anything. The original "why?" still buzzes in my head.

Does sensory information from my hand on one side get pulled somehow towards its destination in contralateral thalamus and somatosensory cortex, as if by tropism? Starting roughly in the ninth week of gestation, does a right brain start to push a pyramidal tract towards the left spinal cord? A mature axon has its own, often very, very long axis, hence the anatomical term *axon*. But, in the development of pathways, axons start as nubbins. They lengthen under influences acting at growth cones at the tips of axons. When fibers arrive at the midline, we can read about their molecularly determined fates. What determines the determinism?

An elegant study, published in 1983 (Lumsden and Davies), depicts phenomena that are anything but straightforward. In the mouse, the

---

trigeminal ganglion appears on the ninth embryonic day (E9); by the tenth day (E10), roughly 1,200 axonal tendrils extend from the ganglion towards the maxilla of the murine face (five percent of the total at E13), but they don't reach the maxillary "whisker field" until the twelfth day (E12).

The authors' several experiments called for explants of ganglionic tissue from days E10 and E11 to be co-cultured with explants from the face and from an inappropriate target, a forelimb bud. All explants were of the same embryonic age. Exquisitely created, little wells in culture dishes held the samples of tissue; the distance between explants in a dish was the distance between the trigeminal ganglion and the whisker field. Cultures incubated for 48 hours. The authors wondered where ganglionic tendrils (called neurites) would head and how they would travel to their destination.

A first experiment found: if ganglionic explant cultures just by itself with no other wells in the dish, no neurites form. The authors kept looking for 72 hours after the 48 hours of culture time.

A second experiment found: if the ganglionic well sits between a well containing forelimb bud and another containing face, neurites extend to the facial well directly. Divide the space around the ganglionic well into four parts: a quadrant facing the facial well, a quadrant facing the forelimb-bud well, then two others above and below. The neurites extend only to the first of the four quadrants, like a dead-straight, center-of-the-cup putt in golf. Neurites don't head to the forelimb bud well, period.

A third experiment found: if you set up three wells with facial extract to the far left, then two ganglionic wells next to each other in a line, then neurites from the further-away ganglionic well (further away from the facial well, only in the quadrant facing the facial well, despite the fact that the distance between the distant well and the face is now doubled) exceeds the number of neurites that form in the near ganglionic well in its quadrant facing away from the facial well. As long as you face the face, neurites head there.

A fourth experiment found: if you culture E12, not E10 or E11, ganglionic extract together with facial and forelimb wells, then neurites extend to the forelimb well–which is without precedent in this study. Neurites of the E12 extract that extend to the facial well do so like breaking putts entering from the top and bottom of the proverbial cup, but there are still neurites that straight putt to the facial well in the quadrant facing the face.

There's more to the paper, but we're in a position to consider its essentials.

In anatomy class, we're used to looking at a structure like the trigeminal ganglion, then we utter tediously, *this* is the trigeminal ganglion. How does a person know? Well, it looks like the trigeminal ganglion. It's located in the right place, so what else could it be? Statements about the right place have much developmental neuroscience behind them, and it's not irrelevant to remind ourselves that, like an annelid worm, we're composed of metameric segments to start. Then, location along the anterior-posterior axis determines differential function. Another way of saying the same thing is: there's segment-specific identity. One could make the argument that segment-specific neurites heading to face make sense, because the rhombomere in question is not at the level of the forelimb. It's at the level of face. We avoid saying that the axon "knows" to go the whisker field, because it doesn't know any such thing. Segmental identity is like a plan already in place before any neurites appear in the first place.

The manner in which neurites head to their target is direct, by shortest apparent route, but travel differs depending on the day. The authors hypothesized some precisely timed chemotaxis along a concentration gradient between wells. The hypothesis still has legs today, as we'll discuss. The paper didn't identify a responsible chemical, but would a hypothetical trigeminal neurotropic factor explain what they observed? We've already delved a bit into many forces at play. Proper chemotaxis depends on the rhombomere. In the absence of appropriate target tissue, there are no neurites at all. If on the wrong day, we have errant neurites. Timing is also key.

In general, chemotaxis changes some random movement or growth into a particular direction; it's a reduction in disorder. But chemotaxis alone can't explain the fated destination of a neurite. There are other considerations, as a widening gyre of papers on guidance attests. To have a fate is quite complex biology.

Beware of the word "complex." Often it means, we dunno.

*

If we think geometrically, an axis is a line without breadth that separates sides, top from bottom, front from back. A neural axis is different. It can be defined chemically as something with volume and content. In spinal cord preparations, diffusible proteins along the midline have been isolated; the first among them (related to crossings) were named netrins. I should be specific: netrin-1 concentrates at the cord's ventral surface along the longitudinal midline, with a concentration gradient ventral to dorsal (high to low concentration) along *that* bottom-to-top midline. What we mean by the midline has already become more complicated than a line in geometry.

Netrin-1 interacts with axonal growth-cone receptors belonging to a receptor family deleted in colorectal cancer, hence "DCC." Netrin-1 occupying a DCC receptor guides axons to where netrin-1 is most concentrated–i.e., towards the midline. The Netrin-1-DCC interaction is a long-range molecular mechanism of axonal guidance, but there's debate about what defines long range. We might be talking about just millimeters.

Getting to the midline is no promise that an axon will cross it. But let's say that an axon does cross; what's to prevent a netrin-DCC interaction to force a return to the midline? If there's a chemo-attractant mechanism, there must a chemo-repellent one, right? Here's where things get complicated: netrins don't attract all axons to the midline (sometimes they repel axons from the midline); interactions between a different protein called Slit and growth-cone receptors belonging to a family called Roundabout (Robo) *also* repel axons from the midline.

Netrin-1 and Slit are by no means the only molecules hugging the midline (semaphorins, ephrins, and Draxin are also there, all of them repulsive); then, on top of it all, there are gradients of morphogens along the rostral-caudal axis.

We've encountered morphogens previously. Recall sonic hedgehog (the protein) and its role in morphogenesis. We discussed SHH gene mutations in association with holoprosencephaly in a previous chapter. Along the rostral-caudal axis, the midline concentration of sonic hedgehog varies from low (rostrally) to high (caudally). The longitudinal gradient, in addition to the ventral-dorsal gradient at any one level, influences axonal attraction to or repulsion from the midline. Adding to the mix: how morphogens influence axonal direction depends on whether the axon is precommissural or postcommissural.

To me, the most important thought regarding axonal guidance has to do with the verb "to depend." We learned from the seminal 1983 study that E10 and E11 neurites move a certain way; E12 neurites a different, less elegant way. What happens depends on timing.

Netrin-1 interacts with DCC, we said. Well, it depends: repellent Draxin also interacts with DCC.

Netrin-1-DCC operates in counterpoint to Slit-Robo, we might infer as a generalization. Well, it depends: if an axon hasn't crossed the midline, the Slit gradient at the midline doesn't seem to matter at all, but if an axon has crossed, then the Netrin midline gradient doesn't seem to matter at all. Much depends on when receptors and which receptors are expressed at the axonal tip.

If we know about Netrin-1-DCC and Slit-Robo, at least we have the basics, could we not say? Well, it depends: where you happen to be along the neuraxis (rostral? caudal?) also matters, and different locations invoke differing gradients of morphogens.

Good news, there are take-home points:

1. Fate is a vague term compared to a statement such as "Netrin-1-DCC interaction facilitates guidance to the midline." But the statement doesn't say anything about the why of decussation. On the other hand, perhaps there is a well-wrought destiny that we have both crossed *and* uncrossed pathways.

2. The axes of the neuraxis are busy places, not lines of simple division. The contents of the midline(s) have much to do with control of axonal movement and direction. Why would there be so many mechanisms of control if the difference between crossing and not crossing were unimportant?

3. How axons reach their destinations depends not only on local factors at any given axial level, but also on their points of origin along the longitudinal neuraxis, since rostral-caudal gradients are in play as well.

9

A Note about Cartography

There are anatomists who go to the trouble for us to display the brain as if it existed in only two dimensions. The value of such a map has to do with organizing neuroanatomy and even developmental neuroanatomy in a Cartesian-coordinate way.

Let's use the Earth in a Mercator projection as an example of a flat map. Latitudes of the globe are all the same length as the equator; longitudes are also of the same length. More importantly, latitudes and longitudes are at exact, right angles to each other. A random line on the map (called a rhumb) can indicate true direction without need to account for the earth's curvature. The Mercator projection distorts sizes of land masses, but a flat map proves useful when plotting a course, say, at sea.

If one had such a map of the neuraxis, we could figure out starting points and termini by x and y coordinates only. If I were a pyramidal cell axon departing the arm portion of the primary motor homunculus, then I'd start at some x,y place, then move to some other, specific x,y coordinate (I'd maintain a position relative to an axon from leg domain of the homunculus), then follow my rhumb lines all the way to my destination in the ventral spinal cord. For any given quadrant and segment of travel, it might be possible to discover the morphogen or other chemical gradients in two dimensions governing my route.

In preparing for this chapter and the last one, it was hard not to obsess over a sentence from Lumsden and Krumlauf (1996): "Patterning of cell types [in the vertebrate neuraxis] appears to be organized on a Cartesian grid of positional information, the coordinates of which correspond with the AP [anterior-posterior] and dorsoventral (DV) axes of the neural tube: analyses of cell fate after experimental rotation of the neural plate have indicated that regional fate is determined along the AP axis before and independently of fate restriction on the DV axis." If a cell's fate in the nervous system (to become a motor neuron or something else) can be determined by location, why can't an axon's route of travel also be so determined, since we know that morphogens also influence an axon's rhumb-line directions?

Recall a couple of statements from the last chapter. Here they are, cut and pasted: . . . it's not irrelevant to remind ourselves that, like an annelid worm, we're composed of metameric segments to start. Then, location along the anterior-posterior axis determines differential function. At that time, I tried to characterize segment-specific identity in the spirit of Lumsden and Krumlauf. Presently, I plead guilty to redundant syntax that may have annoyed the medical student to the point of distraction.

My dictionary says that a metamere is "one in a series of homologous body segments, as in worms and lobsters." A metamere *is* a segment, so metameric segments repeats itself. Here's a proponent of 2D brain maps (Swanson, 2012) talking about why segmentation matters in biology: "The basic idea is that this arrangement [segmentation] is a genetically efficient way to program the development of a more complex animal because essentially the same genetic program can be used over and over—in each segment or metamere." Next, I'll quote him along with his coauthors from 1995; he says much the same thing, but with specific reference to somites of the body: "One established way to reduce the total number of genes required for morphogenesis is the use of segments or metameres: serially repeating units such as somites that share a primary morphological plan and underlying genetic program, although each segment may go on to form distinguishing secondary features." He's not talking about brain metameres (neuromeres) or genetic metamerism (repetitive expression of genes in different neuromeres), though one thinks that he would have loved, in the 1990's, to have proven both. We'll turn to the subject of neuromeres in a moment.

Swanson's work should interest us because of an idea implicit in using any 2D brain map, especially one that has like segments/quadrants in it: to find a way, you repeat redirections along rhumbs, quadrant by quadrant, as if in a Mercator projection. In the case of the pyramidal tract, the redirections would *eventually* point to a specific destination in the body far away, but not at the start of travel. A left-frontal axonal growth cone might position itself relative to some vector pointing caudally (it might head just southward/caudally based on local genetic, epigenetic, or chemical cues), only later to be directed, nudged, towards the spinal cord, after many, many intricate redirections, including the one across the midline at the cervicomedullary junction, roughly where the head transitions to the rest of the body.

*

On the subject of 2D maps, I'd be remiss not to mention Nieuwenhuys (2011). Influenced by the work of C. Judson Herrick in the early 20th century and of Wilhelm His (Senior) in the 19th, among others, he flattened the brainstem in maps of many kinds of fish.

The medical student protests, "oh, why fish, why now?" Answer: because we get to review some material.

In flattened fish brainstems, all that we've learned—about basal and alar plates in the medulla and spinal cord; tectum (alar-like) and tegmentum (basal-like) in midbrain; dorsal and ventral alar plates in the diencephalon; the alar origin of diencephalon and all other structures rostral to it, including the dorsal alar origin of the hemispheres—, absolutely all of that, returns with a vengeance along with an observation that might escape notice in 3D.

Looking at the brainstem in any routine transverse, sagittal, or coronal section, you wouldn't immediately surmise that medulla, pons, and midbrain altogether organize into vertical columns. But if you flatten, for example, the midbrain into two dimensions, then dorsal, tectal structures appear lateral to the tegmentum. Those midbrain tectal structures, now displaced into a 2D map of the whole brainstem, look contiguous with vertical columns that pass below, through, and above the midbrain. Moreover, the columns (four of them) can be divided into more than a dozen segments (neuromeres) from hindbrain to cortex itself, Nieuwenhuys says. Neuromeres stack on top of each other like quadrants along a north-south longitude.

There are implications of his claim—at least, questions—that might change how we think about neural development. Is the cortex (and thalamus, hypothalamus, all of the brainstem, and, of course, the spinal cord) constructed from repetitive segments? Could the basic plan be that straightforward? Do subsets of segments destined to become cortex, thalamus, etc. really evince genetic metamerism? You could argue that all the above is artifact or artifice: you've squashed a 3D thing; naturally it looks different as a result. Does the changed look justify a rethinking of brain morphogenesis?

Maybe.

Or we might just observe that there's practicality in an organized, Cartesian coordinate system, as 2D maps of the brain and the world illustrate.

10

Point A to . . . ?

We've either alluded to or traced the following commissures and decussating tracts: pyramidal/corticospinal tract,

lemniscal pathway,

anterolateral system,

tectospinal tract,

rubrospinal tract,

decussation of the superior cerebellar peduncles,

optic chiasm,

posterior commissure,

habenular commissure,

corpus callosum,

hippocampal commissure,

anterior commissure,

medial longitudinal fasciculus,

and the trochlear decussation.

Aside from the fact that midline crossing happens in all instances, is there another common feature? Maybe what I have to say next isn't perfect, but I think it's worth noticing that if you travel any of the above paths, you depart towards some destination that reflects or mirrors your point of origin.

Previously, we talked about the body's three dimensions and brain maps of the body. Here I focus on how a crossing path gets us from one brain place (point A) to a homologous place or places elsewhere in the brain. You could call the destination a discrete point B–true enough, point B exists physically elsewhere in the brain. But it's a kind of point A prime, a place/places that could remind you from whence you came, even if you've navigated quadrants away.

Consider the *corpus callosum*. From its genu to splenium, fibers pass from one hemisphere to the other such that there's a connection from one prefrontal area to the contralateral prefrontal area (at the genu); then one primary motor area to the other (about midway in the body of the *corpus callosum*); then one primary somatosensory area to the other a bit further back. At the splenium, one primary visual area connects to the other. One appreciates why R.W. Sperry (1961) refers to hemispheric nodes of connection as mirror mates.

In microelectrode recordings described by Hubel (1995), stimuli presented to both eyes in the vertical midline elicited responses from visual fibers of the splenium, suggesting an interhemispheric crosstalk or overlap between hemispheric representations of visual space. The receptive fields for splenial responses cluster at the visual midline, whether an animal looks up, down, or gazed straight ahead. Hubel referred to those fibers as a cement between halves of the visual world. Seeing in front of your nose is bihemispheric. Prerequisite for the task (I tried to thread needle, if you recall) are crossed *and* uncrossed connections. The optic chiasm is a premier example of partial decussation, with its crossed and uncrossed connections to visual cortex.

Though more involved in terms of anatomy, we can think about the superior cerebellar peduncle as a decussation from one homunculus to other, homologous ones. Elsewhere, we've mentioned homunculi in the neuraxis (think about three of them lined up next to each other at Brodman's areas 3a, 3b, 1, and 2). The finer the resolution of our anatomy, the more we see how wiring and decussation organize some or many plots of the body, of space, or of both. The plots are homologous, not quite mirror mates, but fundamentally related to each other nevertheless.

Axons that contribute to the superior cerebellar peduncle arise in the dentate nucleus, the most lateral of the deep cerebellar nuclei. The dentate nucleus is a structure best seen, perhaps only seen, in mammals, and it is particularly developed (it's large) in apes and humans. Its alleged resemblance to teeth mystifies me; or, one could say it's dental, but horribly in need of orthodontia. On either side of the pontine rostral-caudal midline, nestled in the white matter of the middle cerebellar peduncle, in axial section they look to me like two very winding rivers that form the rough shape of parentheses whose concavities face each other.

The rostral dentate on either side projects, via a decussating superior cerebellar peduncle, to the contralateral red nucleus (the parvocellular part of it, with its small cells, but it's the largest area of that nucleus in humans) and also to ventrolateral thalamic nuclei which in turn project somatotopically to motor cortices. Note the plural; we're not talking about just the primary motor cortex.

The caudal dentate on either side projects, via a decussating superior cerebellar peduncle, to contralateral, parvocellular red nucleus; to contralateral superior colliculus and ventro- and dorso-medial thalamic nuclei; the latter in turn project to this astonishing list of places, located all over the contralateral hemisphere (Nieuwenhuys et al., 2008):

> prefrontal cortex,
> frontal and supplementary eye fields,
> medial intraparietal and rostral inferior parietal areas.

Anatomist Brodal (father, not son; son was also an anatomist) teaches me that if you electrically stimulate in the dentate, you can record responses in specific areas of motor cortex, depending on where you stimulated in the dentate. You can even elicit contractions in the limbs with such cerebellar nuclear stimulation. Both observations corroborate that there's somatotopy in the dentate nucleus. But there's more to the cerebellothalamocortical projection than a repetition of homunculi. Brodal writes in his textbook (1981), "These and other observations suggest that there must be a topological organization throughout the entire cerebellothalamocortical projection. This does not necessarily mean that there is a point-to-point arrangement throughout this route."

The question posed in this chapter's title could be edited: "Is There No Point-to-Point?" Do we believe the news "no, there isn't"?

*

If you examine small areas of the dentate in tracer studies, dentate nuclear to thalamic nuclear connections seem precise. Entire somatotopic representations in dentate and ventral thalamic nuclei match each other as homologues. Stimulating a spot in the dentate results in a short-latency activation of a restricted area in a thalamic nucleus, as one expects. But then there's a long-latency activation of a much larger area in that thalamic nucleus. Why the latter?

Downstream in the cerebellothalamocortical projection, you can stimulate multiple, widely spaced areas in ventrolateral nucleus of thalamus only to elicit a cortical response from a small, discrete area of cortex. Or you can stimulate in the dentate, upstream in the projection, to activate a rather large area of cortex. We already know that thalamocortical projections ramify–spew might be a better verb–across swaths of cortex.

Brodal, whose evidence I'm rehearsing, forewarned us not to assume point-to-point correlations. Original point A doesn't lead neatly to a point B, to the consternation of those who just want to know how axons get from place to place. Notice, however, that all along the cerebellothalamocortical projection, there are homologues of the body: in dentate nucleus, ventrolateral thalamic nucleus, and even in diverse cortical locales. All are connected to each other in the projection we've been discussing.

It's commonly said that for every forty afferents entering cerebellum, there's only one efferent fiber. Much, though not all, of the input to one hemisphere of cerebellum comes from the homolateral side of the body. 40x "in" reduces to 1x "out," but the downstream effect of 1x can be either exquisitely focal or of grander, wider scale. A lot depends on how different somatotopies, all homologues of each other, interact–not only in the cerebellothalamocortical projection.

*

I've always wondered why there are so many somatotopic representations throughout the brain. Take just the ventral thalamic nuclei as an example: each of them possesses somatotopic organization, both in motor and sensory nuclei in that ventral nuclear tier. All homunculi refer to the same body, right? Why are there so many of representations of the same body– and, in what way, precisely, do they interact?

I think it would be absurd and wrong to say that we know how. But we know enough not to conclude something that's probably flat wrong–for example, that there's no neural processing that happens between nodes– homuncular representations–in any given projection.

There's a famous analogy that comes to mind, though, honestly, it has nothing to do with homunculi. I'll use it nevertheless, for fun, and mainly because it helps me think.

Imagine that there's windowless room full of clocks and assorted timepieces; all of them work and they all tell time. There are big ones and small ones, a couple of pendulum clocks and few digital ones among them. A person without a watch walks into the room interested to know what time it is. It would appear that she has arrived at a good place for information. She picks up the first timepiece she sees. It says noon or midnight. She's curious to know whether all the clocks tell the same time, and she's understandably curious to find one of those 24-hour clocks to learn the true time of day, noon or midnight. In the absence of light from any window, she has no idea of day or night. She starts to check all the clocks.

You're curious to know whether it was noon or midnight. But that particular information isn't quite the point.

In the famous version of the analogy, used in philosophy courses, it turns out all the clocks tell the same time. But you can't say–it's illogical to maintain–that one timepiece influences the other. You might think there's mutual influence (because why would they all being telling the same time?), but you can't prove it.

I'm interested only in three things: 1. She enters the room; 2. She checks; 3. She leaves.

I'll risk generalizations based on my analogy, though I still have the cerebellothalamocortical projection primarily in mind. There's input into a room. Multiple nodes (all homologous, like so many timepieces) exist in that room. There's output from the room.

We have no idea about noon versus midnight.

Her entry, checking, and departure are subjects for our next chapter.

*

Before we leave this one, however, I'll discuss a case (Yachnis and Rorke, 1999) for the purpose of talking about the dysgenesis of decussations.

We don't know a lot about the adult life or family history of a 31 year-old man who came to autopsy. He had been found submerged in a swimming pool.

We have more information about his infancy and childhood. There was developmental delay: he walked at 42 months, about 30 months late; he started to combine words at 5 years, the approximate age when American children enter kindergarten. He had a congenital nystagmus. We don't have further details about the nystagmus.

At some point, he developed an oculomotor apraxia. I wonder whether the apraxia was congenital, not acquired, but all the same I visualize that he can't generate a saccade, say, to left. He thrusts his head to left to fix the eyes on the target. There's an issue: short-latency correction happens normally with a head thrust (when head thrusts left, eyes turn conjugately to the right to maintain objects on the foveae). But he wants to look left. So the head movement overshoots the mark (to the far left), then he adjusts his head just a bit to the right, to accomplish a new fixation on the left target. Horizontal saccades in either direction are impaired in congenital oculomotor apraxias, often with preserved vertical eye movements.

As a kid, he stuck his tongue out of his mouth a lot. A partial cleft palate had been noted at birth. At one year of age 1, he developed seizures which apparently continued through his life. But at the time of his death three decades later, he had been seizure free for six years.

His gait, we're told, had always been wide based and ataxic.

And that's all we know in terms of history and physical examination.

The original report of the syndrome in question (Joubert, 1969) tells the story of four affected children in one French-Canadian family. The authors traced the family tree back 11 generations to learn that consanguineous marriages happened in the 17th century and perhaps in the 19th.

Our 31 year-old gentleman's story doesn't much resemble any of the original four cases, save for many suggestions of ataxia and incoordination, nystagmus, and various eye movement abnormalities (but there's no obvious oculomotor apraxia in the original four cases). The 1969 report emphasized episodic hyperpnea, which was not a feature of our man's history. Reports in the last decade or so underscore the phenotypic variability of Joubert syndrome. Two genetic linkages are now known, to chromosomes nine and eleven.

The interest in our case is the neuropathology. Here are the highlights:

a smallish brain (1,340 grams) with a simple gyral pattern, but six-layered neocortex in both hemispheres, with grossly normal basal ganglia;

presence of a *corpus callosum*;

aplasia of the cerebellar *vermis*, a key feature in all cases reported in 1969;

loss of Purkinje cells in cerebellum;

fragmented dentate nuclei;

abnormal decussation of the superior cerebellar peduncles, with marked elongation of the rostral extent of the fourth ventricle;

loss of reticular formation neurons;

anomalies of dorsal column nuclei (also, fasciculi gracilis and cuneatus were not distinct tracts);

complete absence of the pyramidal decussation;

and other findings.

I'm genuinely curious how he made it to 31 years.

A study of five, phenotypically various pedigrees (Ferland, 2004) gives us reason to believe that profound developmental delay, mental retardation, and autism characterize the lives of those afflicted by Joubert syndrome.

Given the above constellation of abnormalities at autopsy, the authors of our case report hypothesized an onset of deformations before the tenth gestational week, perhaps at six-to-eight weeks—i.e., at a time of active neuronal proliferation. At post-mortem, the *corpus callosum* is present, so defect onset couldn't have happened after the tenth week.

The maturation of decussations and an individual's progress towards a more fully functional brain seem coincident.

11

The Room

In clinical work, we localize. It's a hunger of mind, like the curiosity to learn what the MRI says. (If we're routinely eager to see the imaging, it's because we like looking at brains; imaging doesn't always provide answers, of course.) One clue that neurology, neurosurgery, or neuropathology is in your future is a capacity just to stare at the anatomy–radiographic or real–for hours on end. Before you're even cognizant of time's passing, hours become years, then decades. But the brain isn't composed of excellent localizations. Parcellate it if you like, smash it flat, bisect it, or vivisect what otherwise keeps it together, but it's a whole thing. It's a single, cavernous room packed with information.

The last chapter's analogy isn't about an unvisited room. My interest has to do with comings and goings in and out of it; the processes inside the room aren't fully known, though contemporary neuroscientists, like the curious woman, never cease to investigate the contents.

We're about to revisit the great decussating pathway called the corticospinal/pyramidal tract, which we first sketched at the start of this first seminar. We've since learned that crossing the midline is highly regulated, whether we're discussing a commissure or a decussation. We know that crossings exist, some just as primordia, as early as the tenth week of gestation. The *corpus callosum* is seen that early, but better examples happen even earlier and more caudally, like the medial longitudinal fasciculus.

You can survive into adult life without a pyramidal decussation, as we saw in the case of Joubert's syndrome. Presumably, uncrossed motor fibers can take control of the body's sides. Other anomalies in that case—the disarray of the gracile and cuneate fasciculi, the fragmentation of Purkinje cell layer in cerebellum and of the output dentate nucleus, and the dysgenesis of the decussation of the superior cerebellar peduncles—lead to the surmise that some prominent decussations, including the pyramidal decussation, must transpire in normal development after the tenth week of gestation. We know as much because certain words reverberate in the ear: "a given brain malformation may not have its onset after a developmental event is completed." What happens after CLOSURE and DIVISION? PROLIFERATION. Abnormalities of decussation could relate to errant neuronal proliferation.

Let's now add a statement from Sarnat and Netsky (2002), that at no stage in brain development do primary sensory and motor neurons constitute a majority of all neurons. From the very start of neuronal differentiation (recall our spherical sandwich), internuncial neurons or interneurons always predominate, Sarnat and Netsky say.

In major sensory systems like the lemniscal pathway and spinothalamic tract, second-order neurons (by definition, they are interneurons) traverse the midline. The medical student is quick to notice that the long axon arising in a fifth layer somewhere in frontal cortex doesn't synapse with a second-order neuron. That axon crosses the midline at the pyramidal decussation at the cervicomedullary junction. On the ventral surface of the low medulla we can see with our own eyes how the decussation effaces the anterior median fissure.

We've discussed much of the above already, although Sarnat and Netsky offer a new fact that's probably true. Surely, there's no more to say.

There's just the matter of entering and leaving the room. The medical student opines: "sensory input, motor output; it's basic biology. The room is the brain; I get it."

Let's step for a moment beyond basics.

A hegemony of interneurons causes me to rethink what the corticospinal tract is. There's no better example, one would think, of a motor neuron than a fifth-layer Betz cell and its long axon. But what if the corticospinal tract is internuncial (literally, a go-between) itself? Read Davidoff's spin on the subject (1990): ". . . we can regard the PT [pyramidal tract] as an internuncial pathway intercalated between subcortical structures (e.g., basal ganglia, cerebellum), cortical areas (e.g., premotor cortex, association cortex), and afferent inputs from peripheral sensory receptors and spinal motoneurons. As such, it occupies a central position as the site of convergence for several dispersed sets or neurons . . ..”

Maybe crossed pathways are inside the room.

The go-between that shuttles between premotor, motor, and sensory cortices and spinal cord (the decussating corticospinal tract) lives in the room. The pyramidal tract is internuncial in one other regard. Like decussating sensory pathways, it’s a shuttle between hemibody and hemisphere.

What about the go-between that shuttles between cerebellar maps to cortical ones (decussation of the superior cerebellar peduncles)? Also inside.

The go-between that shuttles between retinal maps and visual cortical maps (optic chiasm)? See inside.

The go-between that shuttles mirror-mate locales of cortex (*corpus callosum*)? Ditto. We can stop with those examples.

Unfortunately, my room analogy explodes before my eyes. Inputs and outputs to the room depend on the crossing that we discuss. The contents of the room include all things internuncial, like decussations, commissures, probably also reentrant paths or closed circuits or wiring that we haven’t begun to fathom either in our philosophy or neuroscience. The woman who just wanted to know the time goes away. We never learn whether it’s noon or midnight.

The analogy has served its purpose, however. I may not have determined the telos of decussation, but I’ve placed crossing, like a large capital letter X, at the center of my neuroanatomical view.

The Frontal Brain and Language

12

London

Our big story, made up of little ones, starts in England. The year is 1860, give or take. We'll end with the present day.

Chapters 12 through 15 cover some history of brain science.

Then we'll talk about what Shakespeare's Hamlet called "words, words, words."

*

Europeans, especially the British, sometimes double up their last names. If your mom's family's name is Hughlings and your dad's family name is Jackson, you end up being a Hughlings Jackson. In scientific publications, you'll find references to Jackson, J. H. rather than Hughlings Jackson, J. It's a little confusing. I'll call him John.

John married a woman named Elizabeth Dade.

We'll get to her in a moment.

In 1859, when John was 24 years old, he moved from the northern English countryside to London to continue his medical education. In the capital, people were abuzz about a new book, *On the Origin of Species*. Of course you've heard about it, even if you've never read a word by Charles Darwin. Likewise, many Londoners knew about the idea of evolution by hearsay.

John attended hospital conferences and reported for a magazine called the *Medical Times and Gazette*. He wrote about patients with various brain problems–some with neurosyphilis, some with seizures, some with both. I don't know for a fact when John witnessed his first seizure as a clinician.

I do know for a fact that Elizabeth Dade Jackson, whom John married in 1865, eventually had the kind of seizure that we now call Jacksonian. She died in 1876, and people say John never got over it.

John is also associated with evolutionary theory.

Seizures *and* the origin of species: what do these have to do with one another? Let's start with the seizures.

John's namesake type of seizure, first of all, has to do with the frontal brain.

It turns out that a Jacksonian seizure had been described decades before, by a Frenchman named Bravais. John knew about Bravais; he didn't plagiarize. But we don't talk about Bravaisian seizures today.

In seizures of the Jacksonian type, you might see a big toe jerk rhythmically, then the foot and the toes, then the leg and the foot and toes, then the arm right down to the fingers (along with the whole leg), then the face along with everything else, just on one side of the body. Even as the sequence transpires, the person could be awake and even talking. John could look at a case of a jerking right thumb with a tumor the size of a hazelnut in the left frontal cortex, and he couldn't help but think that the front of the brain was involved in movement.

Around 1860, textbooks taught that the cerebral cortex didn't control movement. In Italy, circa 1810, Luigi Rolando irritated cortex and he noticed movements on the opposite side of the body. His experiments were roundly criticized. His reviewers said that stimulation at the brain's surface passed through to deeper areas. His was no proof for a role for cortex in the generation of movement, they said.

Does it seem odd to you that the subcortex alone could drive movement—or that people once believed so? From 1810 to 1860, experimenters poked at the cortical surface or just beneath it, but they didn't learn much. Here is François Achelle Longet, of Paris, writing in the 19th century: "On dogs, rabbits and on some kids we have irritated with a knife the white substance of the cerebral lobes, we have cauterised them with potash, nitric acid, etc.; we have run galvanic currents through them in all directions without succeeding in evoking involuntary muscular contractions; the same negative results were found in directing these agents to either gray or white matter" (quoted in McHenry, 1969). "Kids" refers to goats.

*

Enter a man named Charles E. Brown, who was 43 years old in 1860. His dad was a sea captain from Philadelphia; his mom was French. When he finished medical school in Paris, Charles wanted a more unusual name than Brown, so he added his mom's last name to his dad's. He became Charles E. Brown-Séquard (Aminoff, 1993).

He ran a place called the National Hospital in London, beginning in 1860. The National Hospital still exists today, but, at that time, it had just opened in a donated townhouse. Its infirmary had eight beds; there were some consulting rooms for outpatients; the pharmacy was a butler's pantry.

Brown-Séquard brought a new French school of thought about the brain to London. The French perspective held that the frontal brain had to do with speech and language. Brown-Séquard hired John as an assistant at the National Hospital.

To get more of a sense of the French school, let's think about a patient discussed in Paris on April 4, 1861. I don't know the patient's name, but the doctor was Ernest Auburtin.

Auburtin described how his patient had shot himself at the head in an attempted suicide. That would be at, not in the head. The attempted suicide wasn't successful, not at first. The shot glanced, sheared away the front of the skull, but left the underlying brain intact. Auburtin said that the man's intelligence and speech were normal after the accident.

The patient could speak reasonably enough and was reportedly normal aside from his missing frontal skull. The brain was visible. Auburtin did an odd thing with a spatula—seriously, a spatula. He pressed on the exposed brain: "While the patient was being interrogated the flat surface of a large spatula was lightly applied; on gentle pressure speech was suddenly suspended; a word begun was cut in two. Speech returned as soon as pressure was removed. The pressure thus exerted produced neither paralysis nor loss of consciousness and was exercised in such manner as to compress only the frontal lobes" (Stookey, 1963). I'm stunned how a word out of the mouth was cut in mid-syllable; I'm even more taken aback that Aubertin thought to use a kitchen utensil the way he did.

Auburtin wasn't attempting to show a difference between left and right brain function. He wielded his spatula to show that the front of the brain had to do with language, in defense of his father-in-law's pet theory. The father-in-law was a famous Parisian physician, Jean-Baptiste Bouillaud, who had been talking about the frontal lobes as parts of the brain dedicated to speech and language as early as 1825.

(If you're curious, Bouillaud's daughter's name was Elise. I haven't been able to learn much about her.)

The French school à la Brown-Séquard, Bouillaud, and Auburtin appealed to John. Functions like movement and speech could be demonstrated to be cortical at least in some way. By the late 1860's, two Germans, Gustave Fritsch and Eduard Hitzig, reproduced Luigi Rolando's experiments from over a half century before. Working in a garage, Fritsch and Hitzig electrically stimulated areas of cortex on one side of the brain's lateral surface in dogs–they used faradic current, which induces tetany if applied to muscle directly. Fritsch and Hitzig applied current to cortex here and there, then hindlimb, forelimb, or the face would move on the opposite side of dogs' bodies. The garage experiments wouldn't pass a research institutional review board today (the protocol's barbaric; the garage venue . . . just inappropriate), but the findings supported John's observations about a relationship between cerebral cortex and the movement of body parts.

What about John and the theory of evolution?

*

To evolve, from Latin, is to unroll. Highly evolved activities, like human speech or coordinated movements like dancing or just walking on two legs, don't happen in the manner of a *deus ex machina*. John wondered whether a seizure rolled back the clock of brain development. Actually, in any brain disease, could we retreat in evolutionary time–or: as John wrote himself, could cortical function "undevelop" (Jackson, 1884)?

Here's a story to explain more about going backwards.

One of John's patients was a government clerk (Jackson, 1866). The clerk had been well educated in British schools. From 1863 to 1865, he had four partial seizures, all involving the left side of his body. Early in 1865, more seizures, again partial, involved his right, not the left body. There was a problem with his speech after the right-body seizures. He was "incoherent." But his incoherent speech didn't last for long.

Some weeks later, John happened to meet the clerk again, by happenstance, on a London street. The clerk seemed healthy, not weak on either side of his body. He spoke fluently in a long conversation during which, John wrote, "if he had made the slightest mistake of any sort, I should have caught it at once." But the clerk seemed just fine.

Then the patient volunteered his own sense of his problem, as John describes it: "On my remarking that I had not detected any defect of speech, the patient said that his speech was imperfect 'when anything came on him suddenly,' or when he was not thinking particularly of what he was saying. His greatest trouble, however, was in writing. He had no difficulty in penmanship; on the contrary, it was beautiful. His trouble was that he could not readily find the proper words, and those he wrote he often spelled incorrectly." "To write a tolerably correct letter," the clerk had a strategy. He wrote drafts.

Here's a sample first draft of a letter. The crossed-out words are the clerk's own self-corrections:

> I glad to say that I am going on all right, and I home [hope] to continue to do so. I galy [daily] take a long walk, and do not find the configue [fatigue] as I formerly did. I am aglie agissue agligere to stop and think ~~what~~ how ~~spell~~ the wors [words] are spelt. I can ver ger generly go on verly well in may makeing the second copy.

Here's the second draft:

> I am glad to say that I am going on all right, and I hope to continue to do so. I daly take a long walk, and do not find the fatigue as I formerly did. I am oblige to stop and think as to how as to how the words are spell. I can generaly go on ~~verly~~ very well in makeing the second copy.

Transcribing a passage from a magazine (London's *Saturday Review*) was difficult for the clerk. Here's the original text, which John read aloud to him:

> The man whose mind is entirely taken up with small details, fancies he has a right to sneer at every one gifted with less minute knowledge. Because he can grease the wheels and tighten the screws of machinery he fancies himself an authority on the laws of motion.

Here's the clerk's transcription:

> The mand woos minds is entirely taken out with sall detales, sances he has a right to seen at every one fisted with lest minute nowledge. Begase Begause he gan crease the weels and bighten the schrees of masheenery he sances himself an authority on the laus of mosien.

What can we infer about the clerk's problem? Maybe in his "undevelopment" we learn about how we first develop the ability to express ourselves.

Looking at the clerk's transcription from the *Saturday Review*, letters and words seem put together as a child would do (weels for wheels). Sometimes, there's a drop-out of sense (I don't understand bighten the schrees, for example).

I somewhat understand schrees of masheenery, because I recognize masheenery; but I don't understand "The mand woos minds . . . with sall detales . . .."

With the actual passage in front of us, meaning gets clearer in the clerk's version. But, without the original, we have a garbled message. We have to ask, "say again?" or "write that again." And writing repeated drafts was the clerk's strategy.

Think about where we've been in our own personal development, since the time of pre-school: consider all the trial and error involved. Once upon a time, a child converted sounds to letters. Then she or he combined letters, then words, and somehow, eventually, linked words back to sounds. Especially in the clerk's transcript from the *Saturday Review*, I think we witness him going back to phonemes and phonetics, as if he had become an early grade-schooler again. He retreats as he tries to move forward.

*

When we think about a cortical process, maybe we shouldn't obsess too much about schrees of the masheenery. Even if you know about parts of the brain (for example, the left versus the right cerebral hemisphere), it doesn't mean that you understand the laws that make for normal cortical function. Those laws have evolved in time, and time can go backwards in brain disease. That's what John Hughlings Jackson believed.

13

Paris, 1861-1865

Xaxier Bichat moved to Paris from southeastern Lyon in post-revolutionary France, in 1793 or 1794. Anatomy was his life. He slept in morgues "to be able to dissect cadavers by day" (Shoja et al., 2008). Perhaps infamously, he wrote that "Two parts essentially alike in their structure cannot be different in their mode of acting" (quoted in Harris, 1999). More than sixty years later, Pierre-Paul Broca referred to Bichat's symmetry with respect to the brain:

> It is well known that the two hemispheres of the brain are perfectly similar; if the cerebral convolutions present slight and incidental variation from person to person, there are none that are appreciable from one side . . . to the other. Now there is one physiologic law, which everywhere else [in the body] is without exception, namely, that two organs that are equal and symmetrical have the same attributes, and it would be quite strange that this law should present here a marked exception (quoted in Berker et al., 1986).

Why shouldn't paired structures, like the two cerebral hemispheres, have like functions? Our two kidneys serve the same function physiologically, so why not the hemispheres of the brain?

Pierre-Paul Broca wasn't a neurologist or a neuroanatomist. He was a cigar-smoking general surgeon with polymathic interests, from painting, music, and rich food to the relationship between intelligence and brain size in so-called savages compared to modern Europeans. He helped to establish the Paris Anthropological Society in 1859. In the Spring of 1861, he was 36 years old.

On April 4, 1861 at the Paris Anthropological Society, Broca listened to the case reported by Jean-Baptiste Bouillaud's son-in-law, Ernest Aubertin, whom we mentioned in the last chapter.

On April 12, eight days later, someone asked Broca to see a patient named Leborgne for the surgical treatment of gangrene. There was nothing Broca could do for Leborgne, who died the following Wednesday, which was April 17.

On April 18, back at the Anthropological Society, Broca reported Leborgne's story, which only partly had to do with a speech problem (Broca, 1861a).

Leborgne's illness had progressed over decades. He suffered seizures as a younger man (we don't have details about the seizures), but he was able to hold a job as a hat maker for a while.

At age 30, Leborgne lost his speech. We don't know whether he lost it quickly or slowly. Two or three months later, Leborgne was admitted to the Bicêtre, an institution south of central Paris that was (then) part prison, part insane asylum, and, more or less, a hospital. You can visit *L'hôpital Bicêtre* today.

Bicêtre caregivers called him Tan. Broca writes, "He understood all that was said to him . . . but, regardless of the question addressed to him, he always responded: *tan, tan*, with greatly varied gestures by means of which he succeeded in expressing most of his ideas [as well as an occasional explicative]." Broca added this about Tan's behavior, as described by ward attendants:

> Tan was regarded as being egotistical, vindictive, bad, and his comrades, who detested him, accused him even of being a thief . . . though this patient was at Bicêtre, one never thought of moving him to the division for the insane. He was considered, on the contrary, as a man perfectly responsible for his acts.

Had Leborgne always been detestable? Broca didn't think so.

After ten years at Bicêtre, Tan's right arm became completely paralyzed, afterwards his right leg as well, leaving him bedbound for six or seven years. His vision got worse. Also: "those who were close to him noted that his intelligence deteriorated a great deal in the final years."

The gangrene was nasty. It involved his right leg from foot to buttock.

Broca invited Ernest Auburtin (the one with the spatula) to examine Tan. Auburtin thought the problem to account for loss of speech must be towards the front of the brain—not a surprise, coming from Auburtin.

In 1865, after four years of collecting more cases like Tan's—and after what Broca called a lot of pondering over his experience—he localized a "site of the faculty of articulated speech" not just in the front brain, but to a specific place in the left frontal brain. He did so with a nod to Xavier Bichat (in the following passage, encephalon, from Greek, means marrow in the head or the brain):

> In summary, the two halves of the encephalon, being perfectly identical from an anatomical point of view, cannot have different functions, but the more precocious development of the left hemisphere makes us prone, in our first groping ways, to execute with that half of the brain the manual and intellectual actions that are most complex. Among such actions, one must certainly include the expression of ideas by means of language and, more particularly, articulate speech.

The two cortical hemispheres might not be identical from a developmental point of view, even if the anatomy looks symmetrical.

Across human cultures, there are more right handers than left handers. If a hemisphere can be dominant (as we say nowadays) for handedness, Broca thought it possible that a specific place in one hemisphere could be dominant for a human activity like language.

*

Broca retrieved Tan's brain after death. He didn't cut it up, but he studied it nevertheless. It weighed 987 grams, which is less than a typical normal weight, about 1,500 grams. Overlying the lateral left hemisphere, a cyst pressed from the outside. Broca punctured the cyst, and clear fluid drained out, to reveal a cavity the size of a chicken egg. Around the hole, some of the left brain's cortex felt soft, as if rotted.

Broca wondered about an analogy: what if the lack of articulate speech (like Tan's way of communicating, which wasn't fluent, despite cuss words) was like the state of a young child,

> . . . a young child who already understands the language of those around him, who is sensitive to blame and praise, who points out with his fingers all the objects that he can name, who has acquired a crowd of simple ideas, and who, to express these, can do nor more than stammer out a single syllable? (Broca, 1861b)

Tan's brain had undeveloped, to use Hughlings Jackson's term. It undeveloped such that verbal output wasn't great, but maybe he understood a lot. Somehow he occasionally got his wishes across to his attendants, who (Tan realized) didn't like him very much.

Tan's brain is still around. People have MRI'd it (Dronkers et al., 2007). The brain sat in a jar of fixative for about 150 years, so conclusions are tentative. But the entire left hemisphere, including its white matter, doesn't look so good, and we're not just talking about the cortical hole towards the front on the left side. The right hemisphere isn't perfect either, especially in its white matter. The authors of the 2007 study talk about how the MR findings are far deeper than Broca was able to report.

They refer to a white matter issue, deep to cortex.

14

Breslau and Vienna, 1874

Karl (or Carl) Wernicke, all of 26 years old in 1874, published *The Aphasia Symptom Complex: A Psychological Study on an Anatomical Basis* in what is now Poland's city of Wroclaw. Back then, the city was called Breslau, a major industrial center of Silesia and Prussia throughout the late 19th century.

His little book, only about 70 pages long, was brash. Wernicke knew about Broca. Wernicke's admiration for the surgeon was matched only by his disbelief that speech localized just to the front part of the brain.

Here I'll quote Wernicke, borrowing the way old German books once emphasized important sentences, with spaces between every important letter: "T h e e n t i r e s u r f a c e o f t h e b r a i n c a n b e d i v i d e d i n t o t w o l a r g e a r e a s o f f u n c t i o n a l l y d i f f e r e n t s i g n i f i c a n c e . . ." (Wernicke, 1874). The two large areas are: a frontal part (in front of the central sulcus of Rolando and above the Sylvian fissure) and, on the other hand, just about everywhere else in the cerebral cortex.

Wernicke said that the frontal brain had to do with movement—all kinds of movements, including speech. The second large area (the rest of the cortex) was sensory, containing what he called memory images of past sensory impressions. Frontal brain and other brain parts are connected. Wernicke's book is all about white-matter connections deep to cortex.

*

When I read Wernicke's book, it helps me to think about how listening influences how we speak. Think about an experiment that psychologists have performed many times: listen to your own voice through headphones as you speak, but, in the experiment, what you hear is delayed by a fraction of a second. Gobs of errors start to happen. You might mispronounce words, omit words (if you are reading out loud from a book), substitute words, or leave off word endings. How, when, and what we hear influences how we speak (Yates, 1963 and Hickock et al., 2011).

In Wernicke's opinion, language–including reading, speaking, hearing, and whatever else constitutes a language–wasn't an issue of a single location. He thought about white matter connecting the front part of the brain with other parts of the brain. "I have succeeded, by means of fiber dissections," he says (although others, like J. C. Reil and Karl Burdach, had described such connections before he did), "in showing a characteristic arrangement of bundles of fibers which lie just under the cortex . . ." in the immediate area of the Sylvian fissure.

Now, about memory: for Wernicke, memory images are everywhere in the cortex. The nervous system, he said later in his career (in 1900), remembers by its very nature. Memory is "a special feature of the nervous system characterized by permanent modifications of nerve tissues as the result of stimulation" (quoted in Eggers, 1997). Memories have to link up somehow, and if they do, we have intact psychic or cortical function. If they don't, we have psychic or cortical symptoms. "[P]sychic symptoms," he wrote in 1874, "may be caused by disruption of the connecting fibers involved in the association of psychic elements . . . All higher psychic functions likely implicate the cerebral white matter."

*

For the record, Wernicke says on the first page that he's indebted to Theodor Meynert for his ideas. Meynert, who, it's been said, possessed a huge head on a short body, like a bobble-head doll, had a gigantic reputation (Papez, 1953). A young Sigmund Freud described him as the single most brilliant man he had ever met. We have to learn more about Meynert so that we can understand Wernicke better. Meynert worked in Vienna.

So, we'll travel south of Breslau to the Austro-Hungarian empire. Wernicke spent six months in Vienna, capital of the empire, at some point between 1871 and the publication of his book.

*

Of the 7,526 students enrolled at the University of Vienna in 1874, about 1,000 attended medical school, according to an eye-witness report that year in *The British Medical Journal*. At that time, it seems students actually wanted to attend class (streaming video occurred later in history, as we know). At least five days a week, someone named Brücke, a physiologist, lectured in a room too small for his crowd of 885 medical students, so one needed a ticket to enter.

A 70-ish year-old man with Victorian muttonchops, named Rokitansky, ran the school. Meynert, with his massive head, held courses about the brain that were "unrivaled . . . probably unique in Europe," according to the British visitor (Anonymous, 1874). There were other big names in Vienna. Billroth, a surgeon, worked at the nearby Vienna General Hospital, removing whole stomachs to treat gastric cancer; he taught 509 students besides.

Rokitansky prided himself that the University of Vienna taught histology, then a relatively new discipline in German-speaking schools. Histology, from the Greek, is the study of *histos*, which is a web, mast, or a beam—that is, histology is the study of microscopically small webs, masts, and beams.

Theodor Meynert learned two important things histologically.

First, not all cerebral cortex looks the same. He hand-sliced cortex with a razor, fixed his material in alcohol, and stained it with either carmine or gold (Seitelberger, 1997). When he compared slices of cortex from different areas, he saw differences in layers of cortical cells. His brain slices were crude.

Later, in Berlin, Korbinian Brodmann identified 44 cortical areas, differentiated by layering discerned by microscope, in papers published from 1903 to 1909. (There's controversy over the final tally of all Brodmann's areas—some say there are 52; some say areas 13-16 and 48-51 don't exist [Olry and Haines, 2010].) In Vienna, Constantin von Economo described

109 areas in 1929. Back in Germany, the husband-and-wife team of Cécile and Oskar Vogt had the number as high as the 200's in 1919. Some people complain that looking microscopically for sharp boundaries in cortex can be taken "to absurd lengths" (Carpenter and Sutin, 1983).

Sure. A lot of education is absurd. But I have a question: if grey matter isn't all the same, can the same be said of white matter?

Here is Meynert's second observation at his microscope: subcortical white matter tracts are of different types, too. Fiber destinations distinguished the types. There are fibers that project to places like the spinal cord . . . or, fibers that connect the two hemispheres from left to right and vice versa . . . or, fibers that connect cortical areas within a single hemisphere. At very least, there are three types. Meynert wrote about cortex and white matter as if describing the whole earth as a nervous network, with "colonies of living beings, capable of consciousness, connected with each other with feeling threads and grasping tentacles, and controlling their image of the world." Wernicke also noticed fibers, especially what he called a spider's web, full of filaments, in the area of Sylvian fissure.

*

Getting back to Wernicke and language: he describes a second kind of speech disturbance, second only to Broca's descriptions. If you read Wernicke's cases (ten of them), you'd find it odd that a language problem associated with focally damaged cortex can't quite be found (Mathews et al., 1994). Maybe his first case is the purest example of what he wants to describe. But she got better before anyone could look at her brain.

Her name was Suzanne Adam. She was fifty-nine years old, a widow with one son. She looked frail. On March 1, 1874, she became abruptly dizzy and she had a headache. She went to bed in the afternoon; she traveled to hospital the following day. When some admitting doctors examined her, they commented about how confused she sounded. She could describe her headache and dizziness, but every once in a while she'd use a nonsense word or a phrase that the doctors didn't understand. She could make perfect sense, but she didn't always. Wernicke himself examined her on March 7 at the earliest, in any event some days after the start of her problem.

She responded "yes" to the sound of her own name, but also to any other name.

When first asked to name some objects presented to her, including a hat, pencil, clock, and handkerchief, she did so correctly, but on retesting she had no idea how to answer.

On daily rounds that followed, she might correctly show her tongue when asked by a doctor, but if asked to do something else ("take the glass from the chair"), she'd show her tongue, close her eyes, or show her teeth. Evidently, she watched how rounds were conducted from bed to bed in the open ward; she mimicked how others showed their tongues to the doctor.

She could recite 14 lines of a prayer without error.

When presented a pencil, she took it in her hand correctly, put nib to paper, but produced only scribbles and single strokes.

By March 15 (two weeks after the attack of dizziness and headache), she improved. She responded to her own name, not to unfamiliar ones. On March 18, Wernicke records the following exchange between himself and Suzanne:

Dr. W:	Do you need anything?
Ms. Adam:	Oh my, now who would anyone say something to me . . . [with a friendly demeanor] . . . But I still do not know . . . to whom I should say someone.
Dr. W:	Is this a pencil?
Ms. Adam:	I do not know now what it is called. I recognize it very well. I have already swelled middle [that's my translation, your guess is as good as mine] with it . . . I know very well how it really comes to be called. I cannot remember it.

Next, she identified a clock (a clock on the wall, I think), sort of:

Ms. Adam:	A watch (speaking quietly) . . . a pocket . . . (speaking more loudly) . . . a pocket watch . . . a very fine one.

As said, there's no brain to study in Ms. Adam's case. After she got better, I guess she went home.

Wernicke does provide details about brains at autopsy in four of his ten patients. The cortical problem in those brains couldn't be called precise. In three cases, the temporal lobe in the left brain was involved in a big way–basically, there was damage more behind the central sulcus than in front of it. The fourth case involved an impressive abscess that occupied most of the left temporal lobe.

*

To find a more exquisite single case, we should head back to Vienna, to a basement library of the Billroth House of the Viennese Society of Physicians.

In 1992, someone happened upon a mis-shelved volume of the *Medical Yearbook of the House of the Imperial and Royal Society of Physicians in Vienna* from 1866. In that particular volume, there's a case report by Theodor Meynert (Whitaker and Etlinger, 1993). Wernicke doesn't mention any such paper in his book.

Here's a summary of Meynert's case report.

A 23-year old woman had a known history of heart disease. About two weeks before she died for reasons that aren't made clear, she experienced, in Meynert's words, "a sudden inhibition of expressive speech" without weakness on either side of her body. Her words came out strangely: a "hand" was a "yellow," for example. It wasn't a yellow hand, just a "yellow."

At autopsy, she had just one small area where cortex had infarcted, in the left brain, in the temporal lobe, in the area of the Sylvian fissure, not towards the front of the brain but, instead, far behind the central sulcus. The rest of the brain was fine, but maybe the white matter underneath the cortex didn't look so good. The report didn't say exactly.

*

After 1874, one really can't talk about brain function without thinking about grey and white matter together.

15

Leipzig, 1898

Paul Emil Flechsig of Leipzig, Germany is upset. In 1901, he's annoyed at someone who didn't use the correct Flechsigian brain diagrams, published in 1898:

> . . . useless. They are neither copies of my drawings of 1898 . . . nor of any other illustrations whatever that have been published by me. They are simply of the nature of misconceptions . . . incomplete . . . [they] can only lead to confusion (Flechsig, 1901).

What was so important about his own drawings? For one thing, they have to do with white matter in relation to the cortex.

Flechsig studied full-term infant brains pathologically; we don't how or why the babies died. He noticed that some, not all, of the white matter beneath the cortex was visible to the naked eye. If white matter is visible to the naked eye, it doesn't mean that it has become fully mature.

We expect human brains to get more complex in post-natal development, because babies do less than adults. Newborns don't talk in full sentences and they don't tell lies. But what's the significance of areas "invested with medullary substance [white matter]"? Of note, large areas of the cortical surface *aren't* invested with white matter/medullary substance at birth.

Let Flechsig speak for himself: primordial zones invested with medullary substance contain "the points of entrance of all the channels conveying sensory impressions to the cortex . . . The individual sensory areas are separated from one another by wide tracts of cortex . . . in which sensory fibers cannot be followed up."

*

Let's think about his observation for a moment. We learn about the world through the five basic senses:

HEARING
SIGHT
SMELL
TASTE
TOUCH

Are they separate? If they are, how do we hold something, look at it, sniff it, bite into it, and even listen to it, to decide that–say–it's a crisp apple? It makes some sense that you don't exactly taste what you hear–so maybe those two senses could be called separate. But I like crisp apples, not soft ones–they sound and taste better to me. You might have a different preference in apples.

According to Flechsig, the brain in humans has particular points of entry into that brain for hearing, sight, and so on, like five people entering a building through different doors. The five people never exactly meet; they never shake hands (in terms of person-to-person, direct axonal connections). If those people had names, they might be:

CRISP
RED
FRESH
SWEET
FIRM

Newborns don't bite into crisp apples, so what am I talking about? Hang on. What about this set of people?

COO
BROWN EYES

FLOWERY
MILKY
SOFT

How do you get from those names or sensations to an idea of mother? An idea of mom has to be put together somehow, probably not randomly.

*

For years, Paul Emil Flechsig lived in a cottage behind his clinic on the grounds of the University of Leipzig. When he retired, he said he owned the cottage, and he refused to leave. The university evicted him.

*

At very least, portions of the human cortex invested with white matter at birth have to do with our five senses. With that knowledge alone, we're in a position to brood–not skim–over very professorial material like this:

> In accordance with the principle of Flechsig (which is applicable to man and the other primates but not to subprimate forms), the primary projection areas now send their connexions primarily to the immediately adjacent association cortex (parakoniocortex); the long connections (either within a hemisphere or between hemispheres) between different cortical regions take place predominantly between parts of the association cortex (Geschwind, 1974).

I'll end our historical excursion now. My next job is systematically to unpack the above passage by Norman Geschwind, who died in 1984 in his office (so legend attests) at the too-young age of 58.

I'll need the next two chapters to do my work. By the way, his reference to Flechsig is the tip of a proverbial iceberg, because we'll need to revisit Jacksonian undevelopment, Broca's hardly original interest in the frontal brain (Bouillaud and Aubertin entertained the idea well before he did), Wernicke and his Meynert-inspired interest in subcortical connections, and the irascible, evicted Flechsig just to understand the implications of Geschwind's single, very dense sentence.

16

Sound

Let's start with the sound of the apple.

Over years of teaching, I've given the auditory pathway embarrassingly short shrift. Now is an opportunity to make some amends.

Since communication by sound antedates written text of any kind in history, a discussion of language should attend, carefully, to hearing.

There's a more personal motivation, separate from my prep for this second seminar. In recent years, I've tried to pick up languages after a long hiatus. It's been observed that a problem in understanding foreign speech is, in no small part, a problem in actually hearing speech. A.R. Luria explains that a person who doesn't know a foreign language not only does not understand it, but also, in effect, she or he doesn't *hear* it–i.e., does not "systematize the sounds of speech." Instead, what's heard is just a stream, endlessly meaningless it often seems, of sounds (Luria, 1980).

Can that person "hear"?

*

Transduction of sound in air to action potentials happens at the hair cell, the specialized mechanoreceptor involved both in the cochlear and vestibular functions of cranial nerve VIII. If you're in search of a simple analogy to understand the cochlea, you'd profit from Nolte (1999), who himself borrowed from a 1975 textbook.

Imagine a cylinder open on both ends. The open ends are covered by pliant membranes—on the top, an *oval* window, on top of which the *stapes* sits; on the bottom, a *round* window.

In the middle of the cylinder there's a third membrane, also pliant. This middle membrane has an opening on one end, where the membrane would otherwise attach to the inside of the cylinder. That hole we'll call the *helicotrema*, which is a conduit between upper and lower halves of the cylinder's interior. Both the upper and lower halves are filled with one type of lymphatic fluid.

Populate the middle membrane with hair cells along its entire length.

Next comes the interesting, if surreal part of the exercise: imagine a dramatic elongation of the cylinder along its horizontal axis, with the *helicotrema* at the apex of the elongation. The basic compartments are all present as you elongate: upper half (*scala vestibuli*, contiguous with the vestibular apparatus), lower half (*scala tympani*, which is in contact with the second tympanic membrane—i.e., the round window), and our middle membrane. Coil up what you've created; you've constructed an elementary cochlea, which now resembles a snail's shell.

An apple crunch, at 60 or so crisp decibels, causes stapes to push and pull at the oval window. Both the middle membrane and round window will also move, because lymphatic fluid in the cylinder (so-called perilymph, similar in composition to sodium-rich cerebrospinal fluid) moves in response to action at the oval window. Push at the oval window; there will be initial downward displacement of the middle membrane, and a bulge outward at the round window. Perilymph circulates from the cylinder's upper half to its lower half via the *helicotrema*. With more pushing and pulling at the oval window, the middle membrane deforms as if a wave runs through it.

The middle membrane, which we have populated with hair cells, is a simplification. The term refers collectively to all the structures and contents of the *scala media*, or membranous labyrinth, including outer and inner hair cells in the Organ of Corti. The *scala media*, in fact, is a third compartment in our model, different from the *scalae vestibuli* and *tympani*. It's filled with endolymph rather than perilymph. Endolymph is potassium rich, like the chemical composition *inside* cells of the body.

There's sanity to the simplification, however: when we think of the *scala media* as a single, long middle membrane, we begin to understand tonotopic or cochleotopic organization. Hair cell transduction and cochlear nerve transmission that result from sounds at particular frequencies depend on the location of hair cells on the elongated middle membrane.

*

Sensory afferents to the brain have ganglia; in the case of the cochlear division of cranial nerve VIII, it's the spiral ganglion, the location of cell bodies of primary auditory afferents. Cochlear fibers of cranial nerve VIII– let's discuss the left one–enter the brainstem at the left pontomedullary junction; they head to one of two left cochlear nuclei (one dorsal, one ventral) which drape over the lateral edge of the left inferior cerebellar peduncle. Second-order neurons arise from the left cochlear nuclei. Their axons head to the left superior olivary nucleus, which sits atop the upper/ rostral end of the left facial nucleus in the pons.

Nature is always more complicated than what we teach. The first step in the auditory pathway, from cochlear nuclei to superior olivary nucleus, is a case in point. I'll dwell on some details, but they should interest us:

1. There are two cochlear nuclei. Second-order axons arising from dorsal nucleus take a very different route to rostral points than those arising from the ventral nucleus.

2. The superior olivary nucleus (sometimes divided into two nuclei, one medial and one lateral) receives fibers from *ventral* cochlear nucleus as part of a binaural sound localization stream (Pickles, 2015).

3. Some fibers arising from *dorsal* cochlear nucleus simply ascend as second-order axons towards rostral brainstem (we'll comment to where in a moment). Why is there a second stream which presumably differs from one having to do with binaural sound localization?

On many occasions, I've taught that the superior olivary nucleus, a destination of second-order neurons, is the first place in the central nervous system where there's bilateral representation of sound. A central lesion can result in strictly unilateral hearing loss if the lesion is infranuclear—i.e., caudal to the superior olivary nucleus—as if the lesion were in cranial nerve VIII itself. Let's consider the subject in greater detail.

Left superior olivary nucleus receives second-order neurons from both the left (ipsilateral) and right (contralateral) cochlear nuclei. Right fibers get to the left side via the trapezoid body, a white-matter tract that passes transversely in the axial plane; it can be found roughly at the level of the cranial nerve VI nuclei in the pons. Some, not all, contralateral fibers (those that have arisen from right cochlear nucleus) synapse in the left superior olivary nucleus. If a synapse does occur in left superior olivary nucleus, a third-order axon passes into left lateral lemniscus, heading to left inferior colliculus.

Some second-order axons arising from left cochlear nuclei never cross the midline, and will ascend to more rostral destinations ipsilaterally with or without synapsing in left superior olivary nucleus. In other words, there's a partial, not complete decussation of left cochlear nuclear fibers—a situation akin to the optic chiasm (the partial decussation happens at the superior olivary nucleus).

Now we revisit the curiosity of the dorsal cochlear nucleus. Second-order fibers arising from it often (not always) pass without decussation into the ipsilateral lateral lemniscus.

So, left dorsal-cochlear, second-order neurons travel along with second- or third-order neurons from contralateral and ipsilateral cochlear nuclei, via lateral lemniscus, towards inferior colliculus . . . to accomplish what?

If I'm quite deaf in one ear, don't I still appreciate when there's a sound, for example, above my head?

Binaural processing happens at multiple levels at and rostral to the superior olivary nucleus, because of cross connections like the trapezoid body and others—e.g., the commissure of Probst, which is another transverse conduit like the trapezoid body or, more superiorly, the commissure of the inferior colliculi.

The stream arising from left dorsal cochlear nucleus ends, mainly, in inferior colliculus. At the inferior colliculus, inputs from many places converge to process sound localization in the vertical plane, among other complex aspects of sound (Pickles, 2015).

The last paragraph invites a question or two. As a meaningless sound, a crunch of fruit or a snap above one's head has frequencies that map tonotopically at the cochlea. But to listen, really listen, involves other aspects: where the sound is; how long it lasts; who's making the sound; and what it sounds *like*. Isn't it foolish to think that the requisite and prerequisite processing of data happens only after one anatomical site? Could processing start as early as the division between dorsal and ventral cochlear nuclei or even earlier, at the Organ of Corti?

17

Arrival at Primary Auditory Cortex

We've alluded to these structures of the brainstem: cochlear nuclei (dorsal and ventral), superior olivary nuclei, the trapezoid body, lateral lemnisci and their commissure, and the inferior colliculi and their commissure.

I've not mentioned nuclei of the trapezoid body, ventral and dorsal nuclei of the lateral lemniscus, or much of anything substantive about the inferior colliculi. But it's a safe surmise that each of these stations (which crosstalk to each other, across the brainstem's midline) probably processes cochlear input in some way–the information could relate to pitch, tone, volume, timing, location, background vs. foreground noise, or what have you.

It seems a short couple of steps from inferior colliculus in midbrain, via medial geniculate nucleus (or body) of thalamus, to primary auditory cortex. The primary auditory cortex is a primary projection area in Geschwind's parlance and a primordial zone in Flechsig's nomenclature. There's yet another name for primary auditory cortex which more usefully locates where the thing is in the brain: Heschl's transverse temporal gyrus (some refer to gyri), a portion of the temporal, not frontal, lobe. To find it, you have to look inside the Sylvian fissure at the temporal lobe's superior, otherwise hidden surface. (Anatomist Richard Ladislaus Heschl worked at the University of Vienna early and late in his career in the 19th century. Rokitansky was Heschl's early mentor.)

In light of what we've said about the likelihood of processing at each station (not relay station) in the auditory pathway, it should come as no surprise that the final connection ending in cortex, from medial geniculate nucleus, simply is not trivial.

Nor have I forgotten my task to explain Geschwind's thoughts about cortical organization when it comes to a primary sensory modality. But long before we arrive at temporal-lobe cortex, as we trace just one pathway heading there, we really discuss the development of a perception. As we know from John Hughlings Jackson, where there's development, there can be undevelopment when things go wrong.

*

What is a (primary) sensory cortex? Can it be characterized histologically? The answer–of course there's an answer–has to do with appearance of dust.

We're not talking about heaps of dust in a long-neglected place. If I look at my desktop in the morning, with sunlight oblique to the surface, I see a patina of new dust. It's uniform like an evanescently thin sheet of punctate grey. In a desk drawer, I have a cloth and some dust spray. I dust. I'm tidy, but I wipe away the appearance, speaking histologically, of koniocortex (*konios*, Greek, for dust). Dust on my desktop doesn't organize into six neocortical layers. But to my eye looking at koniocortex, laminations aren't immediately apparent either; I see an expanse of very small neurons like so many particles of dust on my morning desk.

The take-home is: there's histological monotony to the appearance of primary sensory cortices.

I read (Kaas et al., 1999b) that the so-called core of primary auditory cortex is koniocellular, but a belt, which surrounds the core, is not. Around the belt is a parabelt, which also is not koniocellular. Perhaps I finally understand what Geschwind means by parakoniocortex. Let me cut and paste the relevant passage for you: the primary projection areas now send their connexions primarily to the immediately adjacent association cortex (parakoniocortex). He refers to what later researchers describe as a belt, which wraps around a core, or perhaps to parabelt which is outside the belt.

The core is tripartite.

Wait. Is the (primary) auditory cortex just one place or more than one place?

Enigmatic answer: Yes.

*

Students dislike such answers, I know. But it's no less sketchy to say that there are three cores. The core responds to tones.

Step back, or upstream, to the medial geniculate nucleus, which has three divisions distinguished (in part) by the areas to which they respectively connect. Projections from *ventral* medial geniculate nucleus input to the core. The belt receives projections from no less than four places: the core, the *dorsal* and *medial* divisions of medial geniculate nucleus, and, only to a much lesser degree, from ventral medial geniculate nucleus. Parabelt receives input mainly from belt, but also from dorsal and medial divisions of medial geniculate nucleus and from other thalamic subnuclei and nuclei, including pulvinar. The major difference between ventral, dorsal, and medial divisions of medial geniculate nucleus is tonotopic or cochleotopic organization. Only the ventral division has it.

Roughly 25 years ago, the core *was* the classical primary auditory cortex (abbreviated A1). Since then we've learned that there are three cochleotopic maps in the core–A1 being one of them. So anatomists today refer to three core fields, all of which are koniocellular, and all of which receive axons exclusively from the tonotopically organized ventral division of medial geniculate nucleus. A single core neuron in any of the three cochlear maps of the core responds to a characteristic frequency with some wiggle room, about one-third of an octave. By contrast, in the rostral parabelt (located on the lateral brain surface, not buried inside the Sylvian fissure; parabelt is part of the superior temporal gyrus), neurons there response to white noise rather than tones.

What is the whiteness of noise? I suppose like white light it has many components that comprise it–we start with tones only, then we construct noise.

At this moment, I recall John's clerk trying to correspond in a letter (in his first draft): "I can ver ger generly go on verly well . . .." His effort isn't noise, not just tones either; possibly, it's something beyond noise, because it has something akin to meaning.

*

It's time to unpack–or, rather, interpret and rewrite–Geschwind from 1974:

In accordance with the principle of Flechsig (which is applicable to man and the other primates but not to subprimate forms) . . .

Paul Emil Flechsig of Leipzig happened upon a kind of revelation especially pertinent to humans and primates. His "principle" is *not* . . .

. . . *the primary projection areas now send their connexions primarily to the immediately adjacent association cortex (parakoniocortex). . .*"

. . . to repeat, is *not* that primary projection areas of cortex, like primary auditory cortex, project to immediately adjacent areas. Neurons have axons that connect to many places. Why wouldn't there be connections (connexions) to nearest-neighbor cortex? Theodor Meynert observed as much at his microscope in Vienna. Flechsig's principle is that primary sensory areas don't communicate directly with each other in primates and humans.

. . . *the long connexions (either within a hemisphere or between hemispheres) between different cortical regions take place predominantly between parts of the association cortex.*

Connectivity, like myelination, isn't unique to primates and humans. When Wernicke divided the whole brain into frontal/motor and, well, everything else/sensory (non-frontal brain occupies itself with sensation *a lot*: think about all the cortical space dedicated just to visual and auditory processing), he thought that connections were so important that all higher functions had to implicate white matter.

From a different point of view, what seems perfectly unique in the primate and human brain is the exaggerated cortical territory between (beyond) so-called unimodal association areas–e.g., unimodal belt and parabelt connections lead afield from the core, and very far afield from the parabelt, as far as the prefrontal brain (Kaas and Hackett, 1999a).

Beyond unimodal association areas, we have what Flechsig called "wide tracts of cortex . . . in which sensory fibers cannot be followed up," or what A.R. Luria (1966 and 1980) called tertiary zones (e.g., core = primary; belt/parabelt = secondary; beyond parabelt = tertiary), or what we currently describe as multimodal (or heteromodal) association areas.

In a rewind of evolution, what do we lose in terms of anatomical parts if we undevelop a primate or human brain? I'd wonder about Luria's tertiary zones, about multimodality.

18

Pierre Marie's Issue

Academics have their testy moments as other people do. Pierre Marie (1853-1940)–who established a neurological service at Bicêtre long after Tan's time there, who was an ardent student of Jean-Martin Charcot, and who eventually succeeded (in his 60's, though Marie lived well into his 80's) to Charcot's professorship at the Salpêtrière in eastern Paris–was a king of snark when it came to Broca's "area." I base my claim on the title of a paper from 1906: *La Troisième Circonvolution Frontal Gauche ne Joue aucun Role Spéciale dans la Fonction du Langage* [The third left frontal convolution plays no special role whatsoever in the function of language] (quoted in Finger, 1994). For our purposes, we can call the third frontal convolution, or *pars opercularis* of the inferior frontal gyrus, Broca's area. But there's debate to this day over whether it has clear boundaries.

Another of Broca's critics, Wernicke, would be subject to similar criticism regarding localization of *his own* area, which we say is roughly in the posterior third of the superior temporal gyrus (in the left hemisphere for most of us). A modern heir to Wernicke writes, "Wernicke's area has no universally accepted boundary. It is usually defined as 'the region which causes Wernicke's aphasia when damaged'" (Mesulam, 2000). That's funny, I think.

As a bedside clinician, part of me appreciates Marie's reduction of complexity to rules that are serviceable and, above all, simple. He wrote in the 1906 paper: "We have seen, as a matter of fact, that the only notable difference between the aphasia of Wernicke and the aphasia of Broca is that in the first, patients speak more or less badly, while in the second they do not speak at all. But in both forms, one finds that intellectual deficit which had as its immediate consequence difficulty in understanding sentences which are a little bit complicated and difficulty with or the total loss of reading and writing." According to Marie's rule for the bedside evaluation of language, we could say the following about cases that we've encountered so far:

1. Jackson's government clerk had a problem especially with writing. He exhibited, just as he described of himself, what modern aphasiologists call *la conduite d'approche* or successive attempts to self-correct (Bernal and Ardila, 2009). He understood language well enough to take dictation, though very imperfectly. Bedside conclusion: probably not a frontal aphasia.

2. Tan couldn't speak, but he seemed to understand at least something of his environment at Bicêtre, maybe especially how the attendants came to dislike him. (We didn't explore Broca's second clinical case, who was a man named Lelong with a very limited vocabulary—*oui*, *non*, *toujours*, maybe another word or two in French. He essentially had no speech. He could not write.) Bedside conclusion in both cases: probably frontal. The hint is that they are both Broca's cases. But how focal is the lesion in either case? Perhaps not focal at all.

3. Regarding Suzanne Adam, I wonder: could she understand Wernicke? We don't know where the lesion(s) was/were. According to Marie's rule, however, the bedside conclusion would be: probably not a frontal aphasia. Why? She speaks more or less badly, but she speaks.

4. In the case of Meynert's 23 year-old woman, a human hand was a "yellow" (not a yellow hand, just a "yellow"). Is the word yellow (*gelb* in German) all that different from the word hand (*hand* in German)? In German, both are four-letter words with one vowel; in both, there's one vowel tone with consonants surrounding it. Her words, Meynert said, came out strangely—which suggests to me that substitutions like *gelb* for *hand* happened in the context of fluent verbal output. Bedside conclusion: probably not a frontal aphasia.

Can one begin to understand why Marie's real issue wasn't so opprobrious as the title of his 1906 paper? Many aphasias look like cases

1, 3, and 4; fewer have features of case 2, except in the common instance of an aphasia, more global than focal, with a right hemiplegia and a right visual field cut–in such a case, one barely needs either a neurologist or a brain image to envision the global destruction of left hemisphere.

*

My intent is not to subtract from lovely analyses that aphasiologists perform today. Rather, I'm interested in the impression of a language problem. In our routine bedside examination, after we've simply listened for a while, we test naming, repetition, and comprehension; we obtain a sample of writing. We look at the penned words. Sometimes, we just want to see if the writing implement meaningfully hits paper at all. We listen to language out of the mouth of patients, attentive to missteps for which we have studious names.

Today, let's admit, we're not far from Marie's pragmatism at the bedside, because we're interested to discover, at a glance if possible, where the nidus of a problem might be in what we now fancifully call a distributed language network.

(I'm aware that a more thorough examination of language explores, for example, the components of Gerstmann syndrome, or the features of alexia without agraphia, or clues to reveal any of a number of well-described entities in neurology. But perhaps a personally embarrassing story will help explain my approach.)

As a chief neurology resident in Boston a long time ago, naturally I wanted to be a fountain of knowledge and a paragon of acumen for junior residents and students. I recall teaching one day about *paraphrasic* errors in dysphasic speech–the word that came out of my mouth was "para-'phrasic.'" I thought I did a passable job describing phonemic or literal vs. semantic or verbal substitutions, etc. But "para-'phrasic'" kept coming out of my chief-residential mouth, until a junior resident, whose look of condescending disgust I recall to this moment, said "oh, for God's sake, the word is para*phasic*."

It's hard to retain dignity under such circumstances. One extra "r," and it seemed my future had already been cast in shadow. At least, I learned not to speak outside my ken. To this day.

I'm neither an aphasiologist nor a network theorist, but I am fundamentally interested in language. I seek plain-spoken-ness like Pierre Marie, but without testiness.

One way to deconstruct—to begin to understand—a distributed network is to glean what multimodality means and how it operates. In the next two chapters, we'll look at two multimodal areas, one temporo-parietal-occipital and the other—more mysterious perhaps—frontal-prefrontal.

19

A Problem With Naming, Part I

In front of me, I have *The Assessment of Aphasia and Related Disorders*, by Goodglass and Kaplan, in its second edition (1983), because it's the book I used in my training. It's remarkable to reflect how often over 30 years I've taught what the authors wrote, especially the first sentence of what follows, that "[n]aming to visual presentation is a universally used test for aphasia since virtually all aphasic patients have some loss of capacity to perform. While it may be described as a visual input/oral output task, there is reason to believe that this is a simplistic view that does not do justice to the intervening processes."

Naturally we're interested in the intervening processes. But my approach is not—I hope it's not—akin to contemporary articles that presume to tell us about the neural basis of object naming or some other aspect of human language. I'm interested to know more about just two things.

First, why is anomia or dysnomia so consistently characteristic of dominant hemispheric lesions? Second, in light of the fact that a hemisphere is a vast amount of neurological real estate, do problems with naming help us understand different locales of multimodal processing? (Yes, I know I haven't yet discussed what multiple modes are involved. I ask for patience.)

*

The Boston Diagnostic Aphasia Examination is a Goodglass-Kaplan instrument with many sections. We'll refer only to portions of it for our discussion. For example, what's the difference between naming based on questions of this type–

What do we cut paper with?

or

What color is grass?

–as opposed to a battery of naming tests that explores seven different categories? The latter is a lengthier, more demanding test; here are the seven categories, with sample queries per category (patients are asked to identify objects, letters, etc. when the examiner points to a picture or image of the item to be named):

Objects:	glove
	feather
Letters:	R
	L
Geometric Forms:	square
	triangle
Actions:	sleeping
	falling
Numbers:	1936
	42
Colors:	blue
	purple
Body Parts:	nose
	shoulder

Is a question such as "what do we cut paper with?" a test of naming or an interrogation about the verb "to cut"? Knives cut, as do scissors. The authors say: one seeks *response* (the name of an item) without a visual cue—that's nominally and exclusively what the test seeks to reveal. The lengthier test involves naming in multiple categories of objects after visual presentation of an item to be named. Both tests are scored not only on the basis of correct answers, but also on how long it takes for the answer to emerge after the requisite neural churning has been accomplished—or, in some cases, not accomplished.

To state the obvious, responsive naming (what do we cut paper with?) is an aural test.

Visual confrontation naming—the examiner points to an image—is both a visual and aural test, since the preliminary instructions need to be heard and understood, as is true as well for the responsive naming test. Results of the two tests in aphasic patients correlate with each other, in general. That is, a problem with responsive naming tends to be as severe as a problem in visual confrontation naming in aphasia. But there are exceptions. Let's consider two examples, one in this chapter and one in the next.

*

A 54 year-old man, whose previous work had to do with ship building, suffered an ischemic stroke. At first, his right body was affected both in terms of movement and sensation. He improved over three months to the point where he could move his right arm and hand rather well, but a cortical sensory deficit persisted in his right arm—and, it's reasonable to assume, also in his right hand.

I hope that the reader has had the experience of seeing and wondering about what happens in strokes with respect to the sense of touch, as opposed to what happens in polyneuropathies or polyradiculopathies. In a cortical deficit rather than a neuropathic one, it's not merely that you can't feel; there's a problem identifying abstract aspects of a sensation. With a pass of an examiner's finger on the skin, can the patient appreciate whether the movement is up vs. down? With palpation alone in the affected hand (with eyes closed), can that person identify what an object is? Place an American coin in that hand: can she or he appreciate the difference between a dime and a quarter, a quarter and a nickel? What if the coin were placed in the left, not the right hand?

I'd guess that the 54 year-old would have a problem both with the visual identification of any coin as well as with its tactile identification in either hand. I could be wrong. But we know from Goodglass and Kaplan that visual confrontation naming was poor across categories. His cumulative score, expressed as a percentile (100 being normal), was about 30. Why should his tactile naming be any different in either hand?

*

An anecdote.

A late teacher of mine once drew my attention to how aphasics explore sets of pictures with no instruction whatsoever about what to do in the test. He was curious about their eye movements–whether the eyes might reveal whether aphasics comprehended what's in view (Locke, 2014). The concept is interesting: to look around, *with* an anomia. What's that *like*? Maybe an aphasic person knows aspects of an object without an ability to name it. An anomia isn't necessarily either an agnosia or a failure to recognize–but in agnosia one can't name, because one doesn't recognize in the first place (Mesulam, 2000). In an anomia, one may not access the name, but yet . . . one could know the object of interest.

I wonder whether there isn't a relationship, in some cases, between dysnomia and (for lack of a better word) a hyper-nomia. If I look at grass, let's say I think of "the beautiful uncut hair of graves" (Walt Whitman in *Leaves of Grass*). How would the poetry score in the eyes of the examiner? Or, if I see "42," what if my response is "Jackie Robinson" or "Dodger" or (this next one is cryptic; you have to know about Bronx, not Brooklyn history) "cutter"? If the examiner interviewing me knew nothing of baseball, I might be admitted somewhere immediately.

*

What if we show the ship builder an American dime, or we place one in his hand, and we ask whether it's a dime? (The question differs from the visual-confrontation naming test, because in the latter an examiner never verbally identifies any item.) I wonder how he'd respond. I don't know, but, again, my guess is that he wouldn't do well.

Alternatively, let's say I'm wrong. Maybe he readily acknowledges a penny as a cent, a dime as ten cents, etc. even if words "penny" and "dime" never come out of his mouth. Do we then say that he knows coins?

The interesting result is that he scored in the 90th percentile for responsive naming. Perhaps if he were asked "name the smallest American coin by size," he'd respond correctly. Or: was his relative success due to a knee-jerk reflexive quality in the answer "green" (for example) in response to "what color is grass?"

He comprehended verbal instructions, but he couldn't read or write. He couldn't spell words dictated to him. He often confused right from left. He was lousy at math (10th percentile).

What modes are involved, based on the clinical information provided? We're not told about a visual field defect or a cortical blindness–let's say there wasn't any such problem, for the sake of argument. Then why couldn't he identify objects presented visually? Responsive naming was almost normal, and he could understand verbal instructions, so why couldn't he take dictation? And, of course, we were told right off the bat about his cortical somatosensory problem on the right.

Lesion localization isn't the issue here; nor is the diagnosis attached to the 54 year-old's case (our textbook says it was an anomic aphasia–a term that has always struck me as redundant). Our interest is whether we can confidently think of an auditory cortical, somatosensory cortical, or visual cortical explanation for his dissociated naming problem–the difference between his responsive and visual confrontation naming.

For our ship builder, sounds, sights, and sensation enter the brain like parts for assembly, with near-normal responses to the spoken word. Listening seemed his relative strength, although other domains of his cortical function went either awry or, more likely, couldn't compensate when a task changed mode–e.g., the switch from responsive naming to visual confrontation naming.

*

Let me remind the reader where we ended after arrival at primary (core) auditory cortex. I'll cut and paste to help the memory: . . . what seems perfectly unique in the primate and human brain is the exaggerated cortical territory between (beyond) so-called unimodal association areas–e.g., unimodal belt and parabelt connections lead afield from the core, and very far afield from the parabelt . . .. Here's a more comprehensive comment from researchers (Kaas et al., 1999b):

> Multimodal integration and cognitive influences on auditory percept formation are realized through connections of the parabelt with heteromodal and supramodal cortices.

To ask "what's in an anomia?" as opposed to "what's in a name?" is to entertain a Hughlings-Jacksonian idea inspired by a book on origins published in London in 1859: the (evolutionary) undevelopment of multimodality.

The Flechsigian tertiary field described by terms like multimodal, heteromodal, or supramodal cortex is where otherwise discrete sensory systems converge in a kind of interference pattern. (My dictionary says that an interference pattern happens when two or more amplitudes of coherent waves intersect.) We can only surmise that the intersection or interference of sensory-data streams happens somewhere, maybe many places, in the second of Wernicke's two large brain areas of functional significance—somewhere, that is, where the temporal, parietal, and occipital lobes meet. As said earlier, exact localization is not our interest.

One wonders whether identifying solitary points of intersection would be suspect regardless.

20

A Problem With Naming, Part II

I promised a second case. I return to my copy of Goodglass and Kaplan. To re-state what we've said: in general, a problem with responsive naming tends to be as severe as a problem in visual confrontation naming in aphasia, but with exceptions.

A 21 year-old male Vietnam veteran, an American, had been injured nine months before his presentation. A mortar shell fragment penetrated his brain. He had a right hemiparesis and a language problem. Regarding the latter, we have a snapshot, which I've edited (this is at six months after presentation, or 15 months after his injury; he somewhat improved over more than a year):

Examiner:	You were in the army?
Patient:	Special forces . . .
Examiner:	What did you do?
Patient:	Boom.
Examiner:	I don't understand.
Patient:	'Splosions.

He scored in the 80th percentile in responsive naming (not bad) and just above the 40th percentile in visual confrontation naming (not good). To be more specific about the 80th-percentile score (unfortunately, we don't have the raw results), the veteran either responded haltingly to many questions or failed outright to answer two of these ten:

> What do we tell time with?
> What do you do with a razor?
> What do you do with soap?
> What do you with a pencil?
> What do we cut paper with?
> What color is grass?
> What do we light a cigarette with?
> How many things in a dozen?
> What color is coal?
> Where do you go to buy medicine?

Was his relative success due to brevity of acceptable answers? A word, just one, suffices in each case.

His writing was as sparse, like his monosyllabic "boom."

He could read, we're told. There's another portion of the Boston Diagnostic Aphasia Examination related specifically to reading aloud. In this subtest, the veteran scored in the 60th percentile–which means that he successfully articulated just two of ten sentences. I don't know which two he accomplished. Here are examples of somewhat complex statements to be vocalized:

> They heard him speak on the radio last night.

> The lawyer's closing argument convinced them.

Here are examples of simpler sentences:

> You know how.

> Limes are sour.

As said, we don't have raw results, so we don't know whether he succeeded with the terse or more complex items or whether he had problems with both. It's possible that the flow of longer sentences, their narrative quality, the past tense of the verbs, or some other idiosyncrasy made them easier to read for him. I can also see how "know how" could cause a reader to stumble into a paraph"r" asia such as "know ow" or "how now."

In the last chapter, we referred to multimodality involving the non-frontal brain. What modes occupy the frontal and prefrontal brain?

*

Among discussions regarding what happens in naming and anomia, I find A.R. Luria compelling (Luria, 1972, also 1973 and 1980). He asks us to consider two quirky questions that we might ask a patient or ourselves–these amount to a blend between a test of responsive naming and of reading. Example one:

When winter came, the streets were covered with _____.

Example two:

I went out to buy a _____.

What's the difference between the two, if any?

The answer to the first sentence completion task, to me, isn't obviously snow. It could be "frost" or "ice" or (in the spirit of a writer like Tolstoy at wartime) "the life blood of Moscow." The second question more clearly introduces the problem of choice in *both* questions, since finding the right word is indeterminate (Luria's word) especially in the second instance. He explains further, "you simply need more information about the particular circumstances in order to select the right word from the storehouse of memory" (Luria, 1972). To me, word finding and naming always involves choice and always is indeterminate in some sense. What color is grass? Well, it depends. Brown is possible, based on experience in the lethal heat of summer.

We're in a position to appreciate a passage from Luria that I'll divide into three parts.

First part: *It would be wrong to imagine that the naming of an object results from the simple manifestation of the established association between the image and the particular unique name* (Luria, 1980). One has to agree. Luria refers to the kinds of elementary associations invoked in the ten questions of the responsive naming test. Naming isn't only a reflexive recall of cognitive connections. A person can perform rather well at such tasks without revealing the problem in an anomia. In severe aphasias, of course, even basic associations are lost–in which case, responsive and visual confrontation test results will correlate, and neither amounts to a good percentile score.

Second part; these sentences follow immediately after the one just quoted: *As a rule, when we see an object (especially if we are not very familiar with it), not just a single name comes to mind, but a whole series of associations in which the particular object is enveloped. When we name an object we must select from these possible alternatives one association, [and] inhibit all the rest . . ..*

Wait a minute. "Inhibit"? It's easy enough to envision a multimodal area as a locale of assimilation, say, of primary sensory modalities which don't connect directly with each other in humans and primates. We basically characterized supra/hetero-modal processing as an assimilation of that sort in the last chapter.

Then there's the word "enveloped." The associations in question aren't localizable to the dominant hemisphere. Recall that Wernicke believed memories to be everywhere in the brain–and who can dispute the possibility? But naming and dominant hemispheric function could be fundamentally related to each other because the envelopes (not their contents) develop there–at least when we attempt to use language for internal or externally directed purposes.

Third part: *[. . . inhibit all the rest] . . . and thus, in fact, carry out an operation analogous to that taking place during differentiation.* Differentiation in the context of Luria's discussion stands in counterpoint to generalization, the tendency for names to refer to some abstract or common property, as in the word "shoulder." It could be part of a human being, of a road, or a transitive act of getting through a crowd.

*

But and yet: there's a problem, and I've partly created it. Recall the analogy of five people entering a building through separate doors.

I said that the five people never meet: crisp, red, fresh, sweet, firm. Yet somehow we construct the name or thought of an apple.

Do we now have to add an inhibition, a sixth sense that intones, "it's not a pear"?

Or, with respect to mom, in addition to coo, brown eyes, flowery, milky, soft, do we now add a stark negation such as "precisely not someone else"?

Is *that* what frontal and prefrontal processing accomplishes? Do its modes include selection, inhibition, and even negation?

21

Frontal Sparing?

Years ago, I reviewed a book by neuroanthropologist Terrence Deacon in which I learned about a syndrome first reported in New Zealand (Williams et al., 1961) and Germany (Beuren et al., 1962). Looking at my copy of Deacon now, I see that I double underlined a sentence about the syndrome on his page 269: "Both postmortem analysis and MRI analysis have revealed brains with a reduction of the entire posterior cerebral cortex, but a sparing of the cerebellum and frontal lobes, and perhaps even an exaggeration of cerebellar size" (Deacon, 1997). Back then, I had poked into the background literature, just a bit. The 1961 and 1962 papers talked about a combination of mental retardation and supravalvular aortic stenosis in children without much mention about their brains; we've learned since that those brains resemble isolated frontal lobe preparations, because much of the rest of the brain doesn't develop normally.

The 1962 paper by Beuren et al. described four children, ages 5½ to 10, three of whom had Wechsler IQ's in the 40's and 50's (normal being roughly 100). The authors wrote a lovely thing about their patients: "All have the same kind of friendly nature–they love everyone, are loved by everyone, and are very charming." A folded xerox of Beuren's paper is still in my copy of Deacon, between pages 268 and 269. Next to Beuren's name, I scrawled to myself, "Read more about this."

Williams syndrome, as it came to be known *sans* attribution to Beuren, is a homeobox genetic defect linked to chromosome seven. (Homeobox: a sequence of genes having to do with embryologic development of the brain and other body parts.) Williams-Beuren brains exhibit relative preservation of anterior cortical volume, but *less* frontal volume when compared to a normal, age-matched controls; mesial temporal volume is also relatively preserved, with slightly *more* temporal volume compared to controls. The neocerebellum has a larger estimated surface area than controls (Bellugi et al., 2000).

To my eye, Deacon–I've now turned to his page 273–goes a bit crazy about the implications of the anatomy: "Williams syndrome provides a distorted mirror image of the genetic changes that must underlie the human symbolic bias. The underdevelopment of much of the brain but sparing of the frontal cortex and cerebellum . . . has given these two structures greater control over all cognitive processes. The effect is to exaggerate the bias to learn symbolic associations, even though the capacity to learn nonsymbolic associations is severely impaired."

Hold it.

Rewind.

*

We've said that primate and human brains differ from other animal brains because of certain exaggerated cortical territories, including multimodal cortex at the interface between occipital, temporal and parietal lobes posteriorly and, anteriorly, the prefrontal cortex rostral to the primary motor cortex. An anatomical difference, so Deacon's surmise goes, *must* be responsible for that which makes us human–i.e., symbolic more than non-symbolic, linguistic as opposed to non-linguistic, proactive as opposed to reactive, charming as opposed to tedious, or what have you.

Says who?

Why *must* it be that relative sparing of prefrontal cortices equals, for example, an ability to symbolize or even to be charming? It's also plausible that the enlarged cerebellar hemispheres in Williams-Beuren syndrome could also be responsible for uniquely human traits. An argument why it *must* be so would enlist the same logic as Deacon's.

I ended the last chapter by asking, "Is *that* what frontal and prefrontal processing accomplishes?" A generous person might allow that I was partly right about the editing, selecting, inhibiting, even negating functions of prefrontal cortex. If I were encyclopedic, I'd add to the length of this book with scads of corroboration, starting probably with talk about the case of

Phineas Gage, but I won't discuss him and will keep things brief. Instead, let's respond to a critic who asks, a tad belligerently, "at the end of the day, you don't know what the frontal lobes do, do you?" Candid answer: in fact, I don't presume to know, but I've got a trump card.

The nice thing about anatomy is that it's what it is. Anatomy doesn't change in the course of my lifetime or of the next generation's; we simply learn more about the anatomy that exists. In the next three chapters, I'm curious to discuss absolute basics of how the brain's lobes connect with each other, especially front to back. The essentials of my review date to Theodor Meynert of the Austro-Hungarian empire.

But, first, what is the exceedingly rare entity of Williams-Beuren syndrome . . . in more clinical detail than Deacon provides? In a report of semi-structured interviews with Williams-Beuren adolescents and adults, several responded to a stock question ("tell me about the favorite moment in your life") along these lines: "Being here [*at the semi-structured interview!*] is the best thing that ever happened to me." We read that "a strong drive toward social interaction makes up an important and distinctive part of the [Williams-Beuren] behavioral phenotype" (Jones et al., 2000).

Even in the context of overall mental retardation and developmental delay, there's something savant-like and enchanting about their conversational language, their fascination with the look of others as conversation happens, their buoyant affect, etc., all specifically in association with their frontally spared brains. Or perhaps in association with their spared mesial temporal lobes. Or perhaps with their large cerebellar hemispheres.

*

It's a bedside test that many clinicians use, especially in the evaluation of a dementia: to name all the animals that one can in just one minute. The number of animals named is the result of interest in the challenge (if you get to 15 different animals, you're more or less not Alzheimerian), but what's to be made of these responses from adolescents with Williams-Beuren syndrome (Bellugi et al., 2000)?

> . . . tiger, owl, sea lion, zebra, hippopotamus, turtle, lizard, reptile, frog, beaver, giraffe, chihuahua . . .

or:

. . . ibex, whale, bull, yak, zebra, puppy, kitten, tiger, koala, dragon . . .

Early word and language acquisition is delayed in Williams-Beuren, but by school age–and especially after age 11–facility with words and a proclivity for low-frequency names emerges.

Despite adroitness with words, visuospatial praxis is problematic: a drawing of a house yields no sense of any building. Even in the verbal description of a spatial relationship (two 13 year-olds are shown an apple in a bowl), responses included "the bowl is in the apple" and "the apple is around the bowl." Yet, in the rather demanding Benton Face Recognition test, in which one is shown a target face and must select other face photos at different angles and under various lighting conditions to match the target, 16 subjects with Williams-Beuren syndrome (ages 8-22 years) performed nearly on par with normal controls, with a mean percent of correct face matches of roughly 93%. Then, there's the joy of simply listening to a 14-year old talking about herself; her IQ is 49: "You're looking at a professional book writer. My books will be filled with drama, action, and excitement. Everyone will want to read them. I'm going to write books, page after page, stack after stack." Delightful.

Back to a ponderous Deacon, now on his page 427: ". . . the hypersociality of Williams syndrome patients, and their intense monitoring and solicitation of others' responses in social interactions, may also be understood not just as a function of modified affect but as a shift in cognitive style, in which an exaggerated prefrontal bias may lead to an exaggerated reliance on symbolic prediction of others' behaviors." Human neocortex–by which I mean all cortex with the exception of archicortex (hippocampus) and paleocortex (primary olfactory cortex)–*and* connections of neocortex to diverse points constitute an estimated 80% of human brain volume (Shepherd, 1998). In medical school teaching today, though a change is almost certainly imminent, we don't address connectivity with sophistication. As a consequence, a throwback argument emerges like Deacon's, one that unavoidably raises the possibility of pseudo-localization: *what if* there's no discrete locale for symbolic capacity any more than there are clear demarcations for Broca's or Wernicke's areas?

Likewise, could disconnection theory as advocated by Wernicke's intellectual descendants mislead us into thinking that syndromes result from clipping this wire or those wires, as if the wires in question were readily localizable? In fairness, both the disconnection theorists and our neuroanthropologist would acknowledge that so-called human functions (e.g., Deacon's symbolic bias) involve swaths of cortex in the front and back, and maybe subcortical structures as well–in other words, dispersed brain locales, not without their interesting connections between each other.

So, how to discuss connectivity in a teachable and meaningful way?

Is language and symbolic capacity frontal? Yes. *H. sapiens* and the 14-year-old professional book writer seem to be cases in point. Language and symbolic capacity are also parietal, temporal, occipital–perhaps limbic, thalamic, and hypothalamic (viz., subcortical), too.

How a brain coheres is the issue.

22

Connectivity I: Hodology

The word may soon become obsolete; to be honest, it hasn't been commonly used anyway in my experience teaching neuroanatomy: hodology (from the Greek, *hodos*, a path, akin to the Latin *tractus*) may well yield to connectome or connectomics. We'll learn, we hope, about relevant tractography by way of the human connectome project, which is ongoing as I write these sentences.

In the meantime, you can Google hodology to learn about hodographs in meteorology and mathematics or about hodological space in psychology, the latter championed by Kurt Levin (1890-1947), whose concept of social connectedness involved more than personal interactions at points in time, but rather invoked bounded networks of those whom we meet, perhaps casually if not randomly, in a long sequence of phases in life. Lewin, it's been said, was interested in "the push and pull of forces" in social contexts which he described by way of Jordan curves (Google that term, too, if you like) which he would draw anywhere, "on blackboards, scraps of paper, in the dust, or in the snow"--curves which his students affectionately called Lewin's eggs or Lewin's bathtubs (Hunt, 2004). Connectivity as a bathtub: *that's* a concept that I'd love to see introduced into neuroanatomical teaching, but I won't live that long.

This chapter's aim is simple, so let me say what I intend in neuroanatomic-ese, a supremely parochial language, then I'll elaborate, and I'll be as brief as I can be.

Autochthonous (local), short, or "U" association fibers–association fiber is Theodor Meynert's term–are intimately associated with long association fibers connecting, for example, frontal and occipital lobes–which is to say, the longitudinal extent of cortex. Long association fibers can be dissected and are well known to anatomists, but the blunt post-mortem dissection that reveals them "strip[s] superficial layers of fibers to visualize deeper ones, destroying their anatomical relation" (ffytche and Catani, 2005).

*

If you understood the last paragraph, go ahead to the next chapter. If you didn't, let me explain myself.

*

If we were to describe the brain not by surface anatomy, not by lobes as viewed on the lateral or medial surfaces of an intact hemisphere, but rather from the inside out, how would the anatomy look? A thought experiment might enlist the following virtual dissection.

Imagine that you hold a gross specimen, an entire cerebral hemisphere, in your hand. As we do in lab, we scalpel cut at the level of the midbrain, so that the brainstem and cerebellum connected to it fall away. Then, let's conceptually remove diencephalon, specifically all four tiers that are neatly separated layers in a developing brain: *epithalamus*, *thalamus* (in embryology, the dorsal thalamus), *subthalamus* (including the rostral extent of the midbrain tegmentum; so, we remove basal grey matter like *substantia nigra* and all grey structures in its vicinity, including globus pallidus and others, as well as some white matter like the lenticular fasciculus (H2), *ansa lenticularis*, and thalamic fasciculus (H1)–the latter three tracts connect globus pallidus to thalamus), and all of *hypothalamus*.

If you insist that your interest is just neocortex, then you could also rid yourself of grey-matter structures of the *corpus striatum* (putamen and caudate), but you spare the internal capsule; you'd rid yourself, too, of all of the archicortical hippocampus and maybe even that nubbin in humans, the paleocortical olfactory cortex, and maybe amygdala as well. What's left is all neocortex.

Now we dissolve all neuronal cell bodies, just them (not their axons), then we look at the white matter that remains. An analogy that I have in mind—as a reminder, this is purely a virtual dissection—is to visualize the frame structure of, say, the Statue of Liberty by evaporating all that we externally see of it: the robe, the torch, the crown, the tablet of law held in the left arm, etc.

In a crude first-pass view, we'd reveal lengthwise beams spanning from front to back in the hemisphere.

From top to bottom in that hemisphere, beam-wise, we see: the *cingulum* (not the cingulate gyrus, because we dissolved its neurons), the *subcallosal bundle* (also known as the *superior occipitofrontal fasciculus*, which intersects the *corpus callosum*, which passes from side to side), the *superior longitudinal fasciculus*, and the *inferior occipitofrontal fasciculus* (which passes through the extreme capsule). For good measure, there's also an *inferior longitudinal fasciculus*, which passes from the back not quite all the way forward—if cortex were present, we'd notice that it passes from occipital to temporal lobe, not to frontal lobe.

That amounts to six principle length-wise beams. The first three intersect, more or less orthogonally, to the fibers of the *corona radiata*.

Vertically, we notice three main struts: from front to back, the *orbitofrontal fasciculus*, the *uncinate fasciculus*, and the *vertical occipital fasciculus*.

From hemisphere across to the other hemisphere, the *corpus callosum* is thick and enormous. We bisected it, because we were interested just in one hemisphere.

*

There's a nomenclature issue that brings to mind the complaint raised against blunt dissection just a moment ago. The superior longitudinal fasciculus—which is very long, and curves inferiorly, heading towards the beam that we've identified as the inferior longitudinal fasciculus—goes by an alternate name. It's also called the *arcuate fasciculus*—arcuate, we remind ourselves quickly, refers only to something that *bends*. The arcuate fasciculus doesn't arch between the putative areas of Wernicke and Broca. To say so is an oversimplification (Bernal and Ardila, 2009).

Then again, the six beams and three struts that we've identified are also simplifications that give rise to possible misconceptions of this type:

From front to back,

> *cingulum* goes from paraolfactory area to entorhinal cortex

> *subcallosal bundle* (also known as the *superior occipitofrontal fasciculus*) goes from frontal to temporal and occipital lobes

> *superior longitudinal fasciculus* (also known as *arcuate fasciculus*) goes between Wernicke's and Broca's areas

> *inferior occipitofrontal fasciculus* (which intersects the extreme capsule) passes between frontal and occipital lobes

> *inferior longitudinal fasciculus* passes between occipital and temporal lobes

From top of bottom,

> *orbitofrontal fasciculus* extends between superior and inferior frontal lobe

> *uncinate fasciculus* extends between temporal to frontal lobes

> *vertical occipital fasciculus* goes between superior and inferior occipital lobe

The blah verbs I use (go, pass, extend) are intentional: I'm tentative to teach hodology, because we just don't know enough yet about what the often-bidirectional connections mean, never mind the little we know about shorter "U" fibers associated with each of these grossly dissectible paths. It's not that the above statements aren't anatomically correct—in fact, you can find them corroborated in standard textbooks going back decades. For me, however, there's a disconnection between a basic understanding of the brain's white-matter framework and any association with cortical function.

Going back to the frame-structure analogy, if you knew the interior struts and beams of the Statue of Liberty, you could visualize the green-hued statue itself as it stands in New York Harbor or, no less justifiably, you could also envision the Eiffel Tower in Paris, since the frameworks are similar and are both products of Gustave Eiffel's consistent imagination (Lidwell et al., 2010).

Put differently: in the absence of correlations–i.e., advanced hodology plus histological parcellations, plus topological reconstructions (since cortical folding is a challenge to understanding which parts of cortex activate either at rest or in a task–note that a good two-thirds of cortex lies within sulcal depths), plus clinical correlations, etc.–hodology feels like a curio of an academic past. I do think, however, that hodological basics reviewed in the last several pages call attention to the massive connectivity of frontal brain to all lobes–which is to say, to everywhere in the human brain.

But even Ernest Aubertin suspected as much when he applied a spatula to the exposed frontal brain of his patient on April 4, 1861.

23

Connectivity II: Projection and Association

What follows isn't a quiz about the one projection-fiber pathway that medical students recall even if they've forgotten all other neuroanatomy. The corticospinal tract, I'll assume, is familiar enough. But I have a question: what is it, anatomically? It projects (Meynert's term) from cortex, but its terminus is not cortical.

A projection fiber differs from an association fiber that arises from cortex in a hemisphere to arrive at other cortex in the same hemisphere; there are short and long association fibers, as we outlined in the last chapter. And there's another kind of association fiber that connects across the two hemispheres; if the connection happens between related cortical areas (e.g., ipsilateral frontal to contralateral frontal), one refers to a *homotopic* interhemispheric association fiber. Commissural fibers in the *corpus callosum* are interhemispheric and, as a rule of thumb, homotopic.

Alternatively, if the lobe of origin in one hemisphere differs from its lobar destination in the opposite hemisphere (e.g., contralateral parietal to ipsilateral frontal), one refers to a *heterotopic* interhemispheric association fiber. We're talking about tracts which either can be demonstrated in careful anatomical dissection or which are obvious, as in the case of *corpus callosum* or the anterior commissure.

Not all projection fibers arise from cortical sites. Let's describe the last mile, as telecommunication providers call the final connection to your house, from medial geniculate nucleus/body to primary auditory cortex, otherwise known as the koniocortical core in the transverse gyri of Heschl. Fibers project from medial geniculate nucleus; they course laterally; they encircle the lateral geniculate nucleus of the visual pathway, then, at the very low border of the putamen in the lentiform nucleus, they penetrate the descending fibers of the internal capsule and ascend due northward (superiorly) to temporal lobe. So, fibers originating from medial geniculate nucleus *project*. And cortex projects back: the final mile isn't a one-way connection, since parabelt connects reciprocally with thalamus—not only medial geniculate nucleus, but also medial pulvinar (Kaas et al., 1999b).

A different example: what about projections from prefrontal motor areas to subcortical sites in basal ganglionic connectivity? For a student interested in the basal ganglia, there's a mantra that one intones in sleep, that a frontal cortical area having to do with movement connects with a specific striatal locale, then to a pallidal one, thence to a thalamic one. The circuit closes with a projection from a thalamic nucleus related to movement back to the cortical site of origin—i.e., the place at the start of the loop. What's the projection neuron in this scenario? There are two: from cortex to striatum and from thalamus to cortex. In effect, the above is an instance of a projection pathway serving the function of an association fiber from a cortical area back to itself.

*

One can teach neuroanatomy long enough that one overuses antique tricks to get students to recall this or that. Consider how I've taught the connection(s) between cerebral cortex and cerebellar cortex—more specifically, left cortex and right cerebellum.

I have a slim, German textbook with good illustrations (Kahle, 1986) which I've consulted for years. Even knowing that some of its information is obsolete, I use it: areas of cortex (left frontal and left temporal) project via the left internal capsule towards ipsilateral, left cerebral peduncle, Kahle says—so I parrot Kahle.

The central third of that (left) peduncle or crus cerebri largely contains corticospinal fibers destined to form the left pyramid, but the medial third contains a frontopontine tract (so-called Arnold's bundle); the lateral third contains a temporopontine tract (so-called Türck's bundle). The bundles of Arnold (medial) and Türck (lateral) myelinate later in development than the corticospinal tract (Engelhardt, 2013). Frontopontine and temporopontine projections end at pontine nuclei ipsilaterally; frontopontine fibers terminate more rostrally than temporopontine fibers do.

After synapsing at pontine nuclei, essentially all fibers cross the brainstem's midline in the pons (*pons*, Latin for bridge, as in the word pontiff, a bridge between god and man). Axons arising from pontine nuclear neurons comprise the large middle cerebellar peduncles on either side. Projections that have arisen originally from left cortex, via right middle cerebellar peduncle, terminate mainly in the right cerebellar hemisphere as mossy fibers, though some project bilaterally, also as mossy fibers, in the midregion of cerebellar *vermis*.

I've taught all the above—and left cortex does (roughly) connect to right cerebellar hemisphere as described. "That's how cortex talks to contralateral cerebellum," I say. *Talks?* Isn't the verb too . . . colloquial? Moreover, do I miss the fundamental point?

*

Based on studies in the rhesus monkey (Schmahmann, 1996), much—probably not all—of left cortex maps onto left pontine nuclei (motor/premotor and dorsolateral prefrontal, parietal, and superior temporal cortices clearly do, according to multiple sources); there's a mosaic of left cortical terminations in the left pons. In cats, distinct projections from left auditory cortex end in left pons in this cerebrocerebellar pathway (Nieuwenhuys et al., 2008). Even some fibers of *the corticospinal tract* synapse at the pontine nuclei, and will descend no further caudally (Brodal, 1981). Corticospinal collaterals map onto pontine nuclei maintaining somatotopy.

In turn, efferent cerebello-cortical axons arising, for example, from the dentate nucleus project, via ventral and dorsomedial thalamic nuclei, back to what we've previously called multimodal cortical areas, including prefrontal cortex and intraparietal areas. In the last projection, which closes a cortico-*cerebellar*-cortical loop, aren't we describing a kind of association pathway linking cortical locales back to cortical locales, as we saw in the case of basal ganglia connectivity?

A lesson to consider is as follows: you could discuss, as we have,

> . . . thalamus to cortex, or
> cortex to thalamus (it's a two-way, final mile), or
> cortex and striatum, or

cortex and pons, or
pons and cerebellum, or
cerebellum back to cortex, or
cortex and other cortex, or
a specific cortical locale and that very cortex itself . . .

and, all the while, projections seem more and more like associative pathways. There are many implications of the statement, not the least of which being a prediction that locales associated with each other will activate together.

In the sense I invoke, association isn't necessarily a wire or discrete fiber. I mean something more along the lines of: actions that cohere in time and in anatomical space.

24

Connectivity III: An Old Paper

When you're wrestling with a subject not for the sake of an exam, but rather because you want to understand more about it (the subject, not the exam), there's a strategy that proves useful on occasion.

Don't assume that the latest issue of *Nature Neuroscience* or similar periodical will yield the insight you seek.

Be different, rearguard, even Luddite. Go as far back as you need to go; find a relevant and intelligent paper whose methods you actually understand and can articulate for yourself. Print it on paper, then weigh into it. Start to think or write, mainly for yourself.

Our problem is how to think about language as an activity of spatially discrete locales. We discuss connectivity, because neurons do connect for a fact, but it's a more and more intricate concept in the 21st century, as we'll discuss in chapter 26. To peek ahead, is connectivity a history of neurons that have coactivated–and may do so again (Gordon et al., 2016)?

For now, what's a connection, aside from a line between dots?

After we arrive at a primary sensory cortex (we've focused on the auditory pathway), what really happens . . . in what sequence . . . or: is there a sequence? Let's say that it won't suffice to answer, as we've heard before from Geschwind, that *primary projection areas now send their connections primarily to the immediately adjacent association cortex (parakoniocortex).*

*

A paper that I appreciate, because its method is straightforward and its writing elegant, dates to 1970 (Jones and Powell, 1970). The authors studied rhesus monkeys. They dissected tiny areas of pia mater off the cortical surface, causing avascular necrosis of the grey matter beneath; there was rather little damage to white matter beneath the grey matter. After 7-14 days, they fixed the brains, sectioned them into 25-micron-thick slices, then stained those using then-established techniques (e.g., Nauta staining). They were interested to learn the distribution of axonal degeneration in a hemisphere after lesions of specific cortical locales in that hemisphere. One could call the methodology quaint, but that's why I've chosen the paper.

Slight problem: the primary auditory cortical surface hides deep in the lateral (Sylvian) fissure in rhesus monkeys as in humans, so the authors couldn't be sure that they wouldn't damage parietal cortex superiorly or the superior temporal gyrus inferiorly in their attempt to lesion. They probably did inflict damage in what we'd identify today as belt or parabelt. Their honesty speaks to how fastidiously they wanted to isolate only primary sensory areas. Primary somatosensory cortex and primary visual cortex were easier targets.

Despite the inaccessibility of Heschl's gyri, a consistent pattern emerged for auditory, somatosensory, and visual projections due to allegedly primary cortical lesions: "each primary area projects to an local area in the same lobe *and* to a portion of premotor cortex in the frontal lobe." Then they followed the paths laid down before them, where degenerated axons appeared after their microsurgeries. If a first, discrete lesion close to primary auditory cortex resulted in white-matter degeneration underlying a larger superior temporal area, then they lesioned the larger superior temporal area. The first lesion resulted, as we just read, in premotor axonal degeneration in specific *frontal* areas; the (second) larger superior temporal lesion also resulted in prefrontal axonal degeneration in different, more widespread frontal areas, specifically orbitofrontal cortex, frontal operculum, and frontal pole (Brodmann's areas 8, 9, 10, and 12).

Likewise, a lesion of primary somatosensory cortex resulted in axonal degeneration not only in Brodmann's area 5, posterior to (and abutting) primary sensory cortex, but also in the area of primary motor cortex. Then a lesion in area 5 resulted in degeneration in nearby area 7 in the inferior parietal lobule, but also area 6, which is the supplementary motor cortex anterior to primary motor cortex. Note that areas 5-7 are not at all contiguous: 5 and 7 are parietal; 6 is rostral and frontal.

If it seems that sensory projections might converge in prefrontal lobe exclusively, think again. Somatosensory, visual, and auditory convergence also happens in the area of the superior temporal sulcus (Brodmann's area 22, with extension posteriorly and superiorly to areas 39 and 40, in area of the inferior parietal lobule). The superior temporal sulcus separates superior temporal gyrus from middle temporal gyrus; it's the first sulcus inferior to the Sylvian fissure in temporal lobe.

There's more to the paper as we'll see, but what the authors termed double projection from a primary sensory area both to immediate-neighborhood cortex *and* to frontal lobe–to frontal and temporal lobes in the case of their study of primary auditory cortex–makes one rethink stepwise processing. The authors seem to follow a single trail, at first. In their somatosensory study, they lesioned primary sensory cortex, then adjacent area 5, but the trail had already scattered to rostral points (to primary motor cortex). They also lesioned primary motor cortex to find axonal changes under the frontal eye field and both primary and secondary sensory cortices–in other words, a good chunk of both frontal and parietal cortices. Their trail was dictated by where axons degenerated after lesions, but what if spatially separate brain areas could be observed to relate to each other, cohere, or even coactivate based on other ways of looking at brains?

*

The authors were fundamentally curious to know in what ways sensory pathways converge. They concluded: "The most obvious regions of convergence are in the depths of the superior temporal sulcus (probably the homologue of areas 39 and 40 in man), at the frontal pole, and in orbito-frontal cortex of the frontal operculum."

What about olfaction?[2]

Recall the problem of an apple. How to bind CRISP, RED, FRESH, SWEET, FIRM? We can start with CRISP.

---

[2] In neuroanatomy lab, we follow a pathway from olfactory bulb and tract to a bifurcation of tract at basal forebrain; the lateral tract enters pyriform cortex (it's small in humans as compared to other animals), periamygdaloid cortex, and parahippocampal gyrus–all of which are paralimbic.

As auditory, visual, and somatosensory pathways begin to converge, connections ramify across cortex . . . eventually towards paralimbic and limbic locales (e.g. rostral cingulate, as we just said).

The cingulate gyrus, we recall, is also paralimbic, a different point of entry into limbic lobe.

The authors cite a transition zone, a simian homologue to area 35 in humans, "part of which adjoins the pyriform cortex and receives fibers from the olfactory pathway," the paralimbic rest of which receives connections from auditory, visual, and somatosensory systems. The regions of convergence the authors identified (areas 39 and 40 in parietal lobe, at the superior extent of superior temporal gyrus; the frontal pole; orbitofrontal cortex at the frontal operculum) also project to limbic cortex, thence to hippocampus.

In other words, they account for FRESH smell in concert with CRISP, RED, and FIRM. Maybe they get partial credit for SWEET taste as well, since smell and taste occupy much the same sensory space.

*

Fine, there's a lot to be learned by tracing Meynert's association fibers hither and yon. What about language?

By the way, isn't it curious that the areas of sensory convergence are roughly Broca's and Wernicke's areas, if we think about the dominant hemisphere?

25

A Note on Dominance

These autumn seminars try to address a kind of question that students ask from time to time. There are factual queries in abundance that textbooks answer, then someone wonders out loud, for example, why tracts cross the axial midline. If the immediate answer is "because they do," then perhaps (such is my premise) there's something to ponder in a non-textbook format. The preceding chapters don't address left-brain dominance for language in most people. I'll limit my response here just to a couple of pages.

*

Dominance is a problematic word (if there's dominance, is there submission?), because one actually refers to lateralization of a function. But lateralization isn't perfect either, because there are ways in which asymmetry dominates in life. I write (as opposed to type), draw, shave, hammer, brush my teeth, throw etc. with my right hand; my parents and their parents were all righties; I kick with my right foot far better than with my left; if I position my right thumb over a distant object with both eyes open, then close my right eye, my thumb is very much off the distant target–not so if I close my left eye (I'm right-eye dominant). Right handedness and left hemispheric lateralization for language go together for the vast majority of both right- and left-handed persons. At a patient's bedside, if I see a right hemiparesis, I'm eager to examine a language problem; if I see a left hemiparesis, I'm very interested to learn if there's a syndrome of neglect.

(Lateralization of neural function isn't unique to humans. I read that there's left-hemispheric dominance in frogs, songbirds, and mice when they vocalize, and that roughly two-thirds of chimpanzees throw right handed [Corballis, 2003 and 2014]. I read with greater curiosity that in the zebrafish pineal complex or epithalamus there's a genetically determined neuronal asymmetry resulting in an asymmetrically large left habenular nucleus; inactivation of the left habenula causes zebrafish to freeze, not turn away, in response to threat [Concha et al., 2012].)

We shouldn't forget that even if a function lateralizes, there are still homotopic associative connections between the hemispheres via transcallosal fibers between hemispheres. In fact, there are academics who *explain* hemispatial neglect in relation to connections between homologous cortex. Right hemisphere (posterior parietal lobe) directs attention to both hemispaces, whereas left hemisphere (posterior parietal lobe) directs only to right hemispace. Right hemisphere compensates in the case of a left hemisphere lesion in terms of attention to right hemispace.

Right hemisphere lesions result in neglect of left hemispace, because the left hemisphere drives attention only to right hemispace. Here's a theory that's been advanced, with some data to support it: by way of transcallosal fibers, right hemisphere inhibits its homologous area in left hemisphere to a greater degree than left inhibiting right, so asymmetry in function results, with right hemisphere dominant for spatial awareness (Koch et al., 2011).

Is there an analogous argument in the verbal or linguistic domain? Left hemisphere (frontoparietal) drives language production and inhibits its homologous area(s) in right hemisphere to a greater degree than right inhibiting left, so asymmetry in function results, with left hemisphere dominant for language?

Or not.

As psychologist Martha Farah has written with delicious acidity in a different context, maybe "the ratio of critical data to hypotheses is probably too low to expect any immediate resolution . . . " (Farah, 1990).

*

But there's no stopping the academic. Consider a last morsel (Corballis, 2003):

> I argue that language evolved from manual gestures, gradually incorporating vocal elements. The transition may be traced through changes in the function of Broca's area. Its homologue in monkeys has nothing to do with vocal control, but contains the so-called "mirror neurons," the code for both the production of manual reaching movements and the perception of the same movements performed by others. This system is bilateral in monkeys, but predominantly left-hemispheric in humans, and in humans is involved with vocalization as well as manual actions.

The ten-page paper from which I quote is followed by 50 or so pages of open peer commentary, not all of which is flattering, as one might imagine. My favorite title in the bunch of critical aftermath is: "A shrug is not a sentence."

It's true. You can't hear a shrug.

26

Metaconnectivity

Our big story nears its end in the present.

*

This chapter about current functional MRI (fMRI) has seen several drafts on my computer, all of them deleted. In the worst one, I talked about terms bandied about today, such as a dorsal-attention, default, and frontoparietal networks, only to realize that subdivisions of these and others going by different names give a sense of a shifting map or one still in the making.

In a slightly better but still lousy draft, I talked about a rumor that Korbinian Brodmann's famous cytoarchitectural subdivisions were based on just one human brain (Brodmann, 2006). It's probably true, as Margulies has observed (2017), that knowledge of human neuroanatomy in the 20th century has been based on extensive study of just a few brains. I compared the Brodmann rumor to the true story of a certain Russell A. Poldrack, who endured no less than 84 MRI sessions (during 33 of them, he reportedly relaxed with his eyes closed), to determine subject-specific, resting-state-functional-connectivity (RSFC) parcellations (Laumann et al., 2015). FYI: individual and group-based parcellations differ.

In a third try, I found myself talking about the biophysics of blood-oxygen-level-dependent (BOLD) signal fluctuations. Recall my story, from chapter 18, about not speaking outside my ken. I won't.

All three drafts are gone; the single virtue of telling a story about them is: we now have two basic concepts in front of us, BOLD signal fluctuation and RSFC parcellation. The acronyms are less important, frankly, than the words "fluctuation" and "parcellation"–i.e., on the one hand, physiological variation in time as the brain does whatever it does; and, on the other, discrete units of neocortical space that have to do with each other somehow, perhaps mathematically, whether or not there are point-to-point axons known to connect them.

BOLD signal (Ogawa et al., 1990; Raichle and Mintun, 2006; Fox and Raichle, 2007) is a phenomenon whose nuances any non-physicist can appreciate. In a strong magnetic field, deoxygenated hemoglobin has a paramagnetic effect, but oxygenated hemoglobin doesn't. If neurons fire, they require oxygen and glucose. Localized blood flow and glucose consumption increase to a greater degree than oxygen consumed. Deoxygenated hemoglobin disrupts local MRI signal; that signal should *decrease* in an area of increased neuronal activity, but blood flow increases disproportionately, as does BOLD signal.

Three very elementary things fascinate me: 1. As one would expect, BOLD signal fluctuates in localities of brain (or in the brain as a whole); 2. You can quantify the fluctuation; and 3. BOLD signal fluctuation is analogous to noise, but not any noise (e.g., not white noise). There are websites that provide sound bites of different colors of noise. BOLD signal fluctuation has been characterized as "flicker" or "pink," and if the recordings I consulted are accurate, there's a subtle, audible difference between whiteness and flicker/pinkness. The latter noise is observed in a variety of complex, dynamic systems (Gilden et al., 1995).

With the above background alone, let's consider how BOLD signal and RSFC are used by researchers trying to describe a plain sense of mental life.

*

Here's a slightly edited paragraph that merits attention:

> RSFC [resting state functional connectivity] relies on the observation that, in the absence of any task, spatially distant regions of cortex exhibit highly correlated patterns of blood oxygenation level-dependent (BOLD)

activity . . .. While the precise significance of RSFC is uncertain, accumulating evidence suggests that regions exhibiting RSFC correlations are also functionally coactive during tasks. In this view, these correlations observed during the resting state at least partly reflect the statistical history of regional coactivation (Gordon et al., 2016).

Note the following phrases as they relate to each other, from the beginning of the paragraph:

RSFC . . . in the absence of any task
spatially distant regions of cortex . . . highly correlated patterns of BOLD activity

In the assiduous fMRI study of just one brain, I'm not sure what Russell A. Poldrack thought about, recalled, imagined, or how his mood differed during his many sessions. But let's agree that there was no task he had to perform, aside perhaps from not falling asleep–or maybe he dozed from time to time. Why should there be RSFC, in which discrete cortical areas look alike in terms of BOLD activity (there were 616 parcels in total)?

What's a parcel, anyway?

A parcel is a bounded area in two dimensions. A boundary separates a cortical area that has the same pink/flicker noise value as some other grey matter region, all measurements having been made in the resting state (Cohen et al., 2008). Anywhere within a parcel, there should be homogeneous noise. (By the way, the story of 2D cortical maps is itself a fascinating saga; some didn't believe in their utility at first [Van Essen and Maunsell, 1980].)

So far, a take-home is that parcels defined by their respective noise profiles correlate across a brain at rest.[3]

Next, think about how these phrases relate to each other, from the end of the paragraph:

regions exhibiting RSFC correlations . . . functionally coactive during tasks

---

[3] "Noise profile" is my coinage, used for simplicity. The technical term is $1/f$ noise, a temporal fluctuation that has a power density inversely proportional to the frequency—that is, power ~$1/f$ (Gilden et al., 1995).

the resting state . . . the statistical history of regional coactivation

Russell A. Poldrack didn't spend all 84 sessions relaxing. In 51 sessions, he was put to work doing a variety of tests (some as simple as opening and closing eyes to command), all of them dutifully listed in a supplement to Laumann et al., 2015.

Anatomically separate areas of brain correlate both in a task and at rest so as to suggest their prior coactivation. Prior coactivation could predict what happens in the future, too. The resting state itself reflects "some combination of direct and indirect structural connectivity" (Gordon et al., 2016).

*

Does it occur to you that we have some redefinitions to consider? A parietal function isn't necessarily parietal; neither is a frontal one unequivocally frontal. And doesn't reference to some combination of connectivities need more explanation? Enter a paper that invites wonderment about a frontal brain does (Goldman-Rakic and Schwartz, 1982).

Macaque monkeys were studied. Two different anterograde tracers were injected into two places, one left frontal and the other right parietal—both areas in the macaque are known to project to right prefrontal cortex (the left frontal projection crosses the midline via the *corpus callosum*). Just to be clear, the injections were: anterograde tracer A into left frontal lobe (Brodmann's area 9) and anterograde tracer B into right parietal lobe (Brodmann's area 7). Two days later, the monkeys were sacrificed; right prefrontal cortex was sectioned into 50-micron-thick coronal slices. Since the two tracers required different techniques to visualize terminal labeling, alternate coronal slices were processed separately, then camera lucida drawings of the slices were superimposed on each other, using local blood vessels as fiducial marks to get the images in register. The authors wanted to know the arrangement of the different terminal projections. They weren't sure that there would be any discernable order.

"Our major finding," they wrote,

> . . . is that callosal and associational axons [associational is
> Meynert's term, used here with reference to the terminal

projections from ipsilateral parietal lobe] generally occupied mutually exclusive columnar territories, and, indeed, in areas of close convergence, columns of callosal axons alternated in short but regular sequences with those of associational input . . .. Furthermore, reconstructions from serial sections . . . suggest that each fiber system is represented across the prefrontal cortex as a map of irregular stripes (Goldman-Rakic and Schwartz, 1982).

The widths of the stripes or columns varied, ~300 to 750 microns. But the stripes–the authors didn't fail to notice a similarity between their stripes and ocular dominance columns in visual neuroscience–traversed all six neocortical layers.

Sometimes, the stripes overlapped somewhat or even completely: "Thus, segregation of callosal and associational inputs in a rule that can be broken." Sometimes, there were unlabeled gaps between labeled stripes.

*

Here's a schematic demonstration of what they found. "1" refers to a terminal field of tracer A from left frontal lobe; "2" refers to a terminal field of tracer B from right parietal lobe. There are six lines, representing six layers of prefrontal neocortex. But it should be added that overlaps ("1212") were occasionally more pronounced in specific layers–e.g., more overlap in layer VI as opposed to layer I. Also, stripes or columns could appear more like triangles. In this schematic, I'll assume no difference in overlap between cortical layers, and the stripes are columnar:

```
11111222221212222222111 11112222111112222212121111112222211 11112222
11111222221212222222111 11112222111112222212121111112222211 11112222
11111222221212222222111 11112222111112222212121111112222211 11112222
11111222221212222222111 11112222111112222212121111112222211 11112222
11111222221212222222111 11112222111112222212121111112222211 11112222
11111222221212222222111 11112222111112222212121111112222211 11112222
```

In prefrontal cortex, there's representation of other brain areas in the ipsilateral and contralateral hemisphere. Gaps could represent projections from other territories not interrogated by the two anterograde tracers used in the experiment. Previously, we looked at one experiment that begged a question about coherence of spatially discrete cortical areas. In the 1's and 2's above, we're schematizing coherence, which is akin to the types of correlations observed in RSFC study. We've concentrated on R.A. Poldrack in a condition of rest, but there's other study of individuals that reveals connectivity quite unique to persons (why would we expect otherwise?) and personal parcellations that blur in group-averaged data (Braga and Buckner, 2017).

We've said that fluctuation and parcellation are the important words. So:

A question comes to mind (Goldman-Rakic and Schwartz hint at it): who's to say that the above, highly schematic, columnar anatomy and, moreover, patterns of BOLD activity observed more than 35 years after the anterograde tracer study . . . to repeat, who's to say that all the above remains static or fixed over time . . . especially in a person's brain that, say, learns a language?

In metaconnectivity, wouldn't we expect something beyond static anatomy?

27

Historical and Contemporary Conclusion

A Classics scholar wonders about how the epics of the ancient poet Homer, recited by heart to rapt audiences in an era preceding the written word, could be memorized in the first place:

> Why does *epic* oral storage of cultural information have to take narrative form? . . .
>
> The pleasures of rhythm are motor responses, they accompany actual motions of the body and mouth. This means that the process of recitation and of remembrance is itself a performance, a doing, a series of rhythmically co-ordinated actions. . . . [T]he preferred form of statement for memorisation will be one which describes "action." But acts can be performed only by "actors"; that is, by living agents who are "doing things." This can only mean that the preferred format for verbal storage in an oral culture will be the narrative of persons in action . . . (Havelock, 1982).

If we think of language as a skill learned *by doing*, then, thinking neurologically, we become curious about a relationship between, for example, motor cortex/cortices and memory . . . between doing and observing . . . between coordinated action and language itself. Action and language are hardly independent of each other, and treatises exist on the subject (e.g., Dehaene, 2009, reviewed in Miyawaki, 2010).

Language as a sensorimotor phenomenon is no revelation: we've always known it to be so. But the anatomic underpinnings of acts that are altogether sensory, motor, mnemonic, emotional, cultural, etc. are the stuff of many books written and still to be written.

I wonder, in retrospect, whether the title of this seminar is wrong somehow: the *frontal* brain and language introduces a bias that maybe only the front matters. Nothing could be further from the truth.

In self defense, I had history to tell that started, literally, in the frontal brain. It's quite a story, and I'll stick with it.

THIRD SEMINAR

Learning the Brainstem

28

Three Choices

Nothing worth really knowing is easy to learn, but there are productive strategies.

This third seminar compiles tactics that I've used over years of teaching human brainstem anatomy. I'll assume familiarity with a basic neurological examination. I've noticed that medical students now learn in clinics and hospitals during their first year; so be it. That early exposure to patients and their problems demands better teaching from the elders amongst us, myself certainly included.

Also, I know that some students consider themselves purely visual learners, but if the reader anticipates that there will be diagrams in what follows, then I'd ask that person not to be outraged.

The written word aids an ability to visualize anatomy in the mind's eye. Such is my approach.

In evaluating a patient, one doesn't want to consult an illustration at the bedside. You'd seem like a tourist with a map.

To achieve knowledge like that of a local: I'll attempt it.

*

When it comes to the localization of a brainstem lesion, to keep things simple, a person has three choices. The problem could be in the medulla, pons, or midbrain.

I've taught many students who, when presented a random axial section of brainstem, can't tell whether she or he looks at a slice of pons, midbrain, or medulla. It's OK. The problem has to do with how we teach the subject, that's all.

Even if you just guessed, you'd have a one-in-three chance of being correct. The odds in a true-false question are better, yes. All the same, a one-in-three chance isn't bad. Midbrain, medulla, or pons: those are the possible answers. Just choose one. If you're right, then you figure out why you were correct. If wrong, then you ascertain how you went astray from brainstem reality.

You've started to learn our subject.

*

Off my shelf, I pull a worn copy of *Localization in Clinical Neurology* (Brazis et al., 1985). It's a book I consulted *a lot* during my training in the 1980's. It has 21 chapters, ten of which address either cranial nerves III through XII; or the midbrain, pons, and medulla; or the topic of coma. Roughly half of the book, then, deals with the very limited amount of neurological space that comprises a brainstem, which is about three inches in length. (The coma chapter deals heavily with brainstem, even if coma often results from bihemispheric dysfunction only.)

I turn to chapter 14, on the localization of lesions affecting the brainstem, which is only 14 pages long, including notes. The old highlighting in my copy has faded–note to self: yellow ink is evanescent, as memory can be. The author wastes no time; he starts with syndromes of the medulla oblongata (the medulla) on his first page.

If you're like the way I once was, you seek the shortest, best rendition of facts, names, and tidbits–all of which you must assimilate quickly. You have zero patience for encyclopedic performances. As much as I still like Chapter 14, there's a problem with the method: it's full of facts ready for memorization. It reads like a 14-page shopping list of stuff to get at the store.

As said, if someone has any question about anything having to do with the brainstem, it's a matter of three basic options. You know that short list already. Now we get to work.

We'll consult two early papers, both decades old (I'll provide the references later). The plan is to think through the authors' problem by entertaining our three possible answers.

*

They wanted to solve a puzzle: *the localization of a lesion that could cause both pyramidal and cerebellar signs in the same limbs.*

Here's a synopsis of the first case in their series.

A 44 year-old man, whose past medical history included (perhaps) a touch of high blood pressure, noticed while walking one afternoon that his right knee was "wrong." He felt that the right leg could buckle under him. He sat down to have a cigarette; as he lit it, his right hand overshot the mark. He was able to walk to the doctor's office, which wasn't far away (200 yards). Turning the pages of a magazine in the waiting room was difficult, due to incoordination in his right, presumably dominant hand. He was examined. All of the above happened within 50 minutes of onset of his difficulties. As he put his shoes back on, after the examination, he noticed clearing of all his symptoms. But they returned five minutes later.

(I have to ask: he was just 200 yards away from the doctor's office? And the office actually added him to the schedule? But I digress.)

His vital signs were notable for a blood pressure of 138/104. On general medical examination, he was overweight, but there were no reported abnormalities. The pertinent findings were all neurologic. He was alert without a speech disorder. Specifically, he was not dysarthric. His visual acuity and visual fields were normal. The optic discs were normal, as were his pupils, including their reaction to light. Eye movements were full, except that, on left lateral gaze, there was horizontal nystagmus with a fast component to the left. Optokinetic nystagmus was diminished with leftward moving targets. His face was symmetrical; hearing was normal, as was his swallowing. His tongue was not weak.

He was weak in the distal right leg; right ankle and toe dorsiflexion were poor. Otherwise he was strong. Sensation was normal throughout to the primary modalities, but he described that his right hand felt swollen. There was reflex asymmetry only in the legs: the right knee jerk and ankle jerk were brisk compared to the left; the right toe was clearly extensor, the left flexor.

Appendicular coordination, gait, and Romberg were all abnormal. I'll quote the findings verbatim:

> The right arm and leg showed a severe intention tremor . . . .
> On the finger-nose test wild oscillatory movements caused
> the patient to strike himself in the face. The patient could
> not use the right hand for eating. Abnormal rebound was
> easily demonstrated. On holding the arms out the right

deviated laterally. On the heel-knee test there was a most severe dysmetria and the right thigh tended to fall laterally although weakness could not be demonstrated. . . . Walking was unsteady and the right leg was dragged with toe scraping and circumduction . . .. On the Romberg test the patient toppled backwards and to the right.

Bearing in mind that this seminar is about brainstem, it wouldn't serve a teacher's purpose to present, off the bat, a case that's not a matter of brainstem localization. I know my students well enough to predict that a handful would protest that the case isn't necessarily a brainstem problem. The authors acknowledge as much: "If first we set aside for the moment the proposition that the syndrome is the result of a supratentorial lesion, how might an infratentorial lesion explain the symptoms?" The tentorium cerebelli is dura mater that intervenes between the cerebral and cerebellar hemispheres (Nolte, 1999); that tentorium is the upper border of the posterior fossa, wherein the brainstem, infratentorially, . . . is.

So, we've got three choices for localization in the infratentorial brainstem.

One approach is to improve the odds. Can we eliminate just one option to get us to a 50-50 chance?

*

Let's think about the eyes first, since nystagmus was the first reported finding, aside from his high-ish blood pressure and his body's perhaps over-heavy mass. His mental status was normal. He was intelligent, in fact. All seemed fine in talking with him, but . . .

A practical thing to do is to notice what's working fine, long before one obsesses over some alleged direction-fixed or unidirectional nystagmus (leftward beating on leftward gaze), never mind the oddity of their optokinetic nystagmus finding.

The eye movements were full. Can we surmise that cranial nerves III, IV, and VI, and their brainstem nuclei, and perhaps the white-matter connections between them . . . were all intact? If you ran with that hypothesis, then you might exonerate midbrain, the location of the nuclei of cranial nerves III and IV, as well as pons, the location of cranial nerve VI nucleus.

Note to self: cranial nerves assigned lower numbers are located higher up–they are more rostral. (Cranial nerve I is most rostral, but it has little to do with the brainstem; cranial nerve II has to do with the upper brainstem insofar as some of its fibers project *to* brainstem.)

Cranial nerve nuclei III and IV are mesencephalic, in the midbrain.

By the time you get to two major cranial nerve V nuclei–there's a sensory one and motor one in the pons–you're (guess what?) in the upper/rostral pons.

Could we say that the localization of the 44 year-old man's problem must be in the medulla, by exclusion of the midbrain and pons, because the eye movements were full?

*

RULE #1, which might be called the rule of rules and the mother of a scientific approach to anything: whenever in doubt or, especially, when you are certain beyond doubt, assume that you are wrong (that you are null); then assimilate data to prove or disprove your null hypothesis.

*

There was a left-beating nystagmus elicited only in left lateral gaze. Presumably, it wasn't present in primary gaze (looking straight ahead); not present, either, with the eyes in right lateral gaze. What does it mean? The authors don't help much: "[It's] a somewhat indefinite finding but one which should not be dismissed too readily." We haven't discussed nystagmus of any type yet: are we, therefore, already confused? Can we say, for now, that something might not be normal with gaze in the lateral plane?

In part, gaze in the lateral plane has to do with the lateral rectus muscle, associated with cranial nerve (CN) VI, whose nucleus is below that of CN V, but still in pons. There was even a problem with the eyes looking at leftward moving targets in a test to elicit optokinetic nystagmus. Is it perfectly safe to eliminate pons from consideration? We might subtract a bit from our earlier hypothesis: if CN III and IV seem to be OK, can we take midbrain off our list at least?

*

RULE #2, related to RULE #1 (as important as RULE #1): whatever you do, keep working the problem.

*

The last sentence raises a reasonable question: what *is* the problem? His right leg is wrong. And he couldn't light his cigarette. It all happened quickly, just two football fields away from his doctor.

Now let's translate the findings on examination into simple sentences. FIRST (BIG) OBSERVATION: *He was weak in the distal right leg; right ankle and toe dorsiflexion were poor. Otherwise he was strong.* TRANSLATION: He had an isolated right foot drop.

SECOND OBSERVATION: *There was reflex asymmetry only in the legs: the right knee jerk and ankle jerk were brisk compared to the left; the right toe was clearly extensor, the left flexor.* TRANSLATION: There were upper motor neurons signs in the right leg and foot.

THIRD (MAJOR) OBSERVATION: *The right arm and leg showed a severe intention tremor. On the finger-nose test wild oscillatory movements caused the patient to strike himself in the face. The patient could not use the right hand for eating.* TRANSLATION: No wonder he couldn't light his cigarette. I'll bet that getting the cigarette to his lips wasn't easy, either. A task with a target was a problem for him, because of shaking or shakiness. More on his right leg in a moment.

FOURTH: *Abnormal rebound was easily demonstrated. On holding the arms out the right deviated laterally.* TRANSLATION: Is there a relationship between these findings and the third observation?

FIFTH: *On the heel-knee test there was a most severe dysmetria and the right thigh tended to fall laterally although weakness could not be demonstrated.* TRANSLATION: How can a person walk with this problem? The authors already told us about a right leg tremor, but this sounds different, maybe.

SIXTH: *Walking was unsteady and the right leg was dragged with toe scraping and circumduction.* TRANSLATION: Are we talking only about his foot drop (see first observation)? With a foot drop, the toe would indeed scrape the ground, despite all circumducting attempts to prevent that from happening.

Unsteady walk? What does that mean?

SEVENTH: *On the Romberg test the patient toppled backwards and to the right.* TRANSLATION: Originally, Moritz Heinrich Romberg's test (he taught in Berlin in the mid-19th century) had to do with neurosyphilis. Let's assume that our patient doesn't have neurosyphilis.

*

Summary of where we are this moment, point by point: 1. Teacher says this is not a case of neurosyphilis, so that's off the list; 2. We tentatively excluded the midbrain as a localization–which leaves us with pons vs. medulla; 3. The patient has a weak distal right leg and something really wrong with the right arm and leg when either of them move, especially towards a target; 4. We know for an absolute fact that there's a combination of pyramidal and cerebellar signs, because the very first thing we read about the case was the authors' interest in *the localization of a lesion that could cause both pyramidal and cerebellar signs in the same limbs.*

I'm not trying to be flippant–and we'll return to the above case. For now, I draw attention to the fact that cerebellar and pyramidal tracts are closest to each other physically/anatomically, and therefore can both be affected by one acute and discrete lesion, either in the midbrain or pons. Cerebellar and pyramidal tracts are comparatively far apart in the medulla. Earlier in our discussion, we excluded the midbrain, more or less. So, by a kind of primitive logic, could we say that the lesion localization in our 44 year-old gentleman must be pontine?

The papers used in this chapter are Fisher and Cole, 1965 and Fisher, 1978. The syndrome is an ataxic hemiparesis. The brainstem localization is left pons, although ataxic hemipareses can result from supratentorial lesions.

29

The Diencephalic-Mesencephalic Border

Since the brainstem as a whole is such a small territory, the argument could be made that all structures in it are close to each other by definition. That's true, but all things are relative. In anatomy lab, if you take a thin slice of any part of the brain, structures visible on one surface often look very different on the reverse side; sometimes, they just disappear. The thickness of the slice could be much less than an inch. In brainstem especially, a great deal changes visually and anatomically in the space of millimeters. Relations are invaluable, however (what's next to what, in detail, at roughly 6-8x magnification, using your mental lens). In the chapters that follow, we'll concentrate on things close to each other at various levels of midbrain, pons, and medulla—in that descending order (rostral to caudal).

We'll describe axial (transverse) sections, with a proviso.

*

RULE #3: Think three dimensionally.

*

An immediate application of Rule #3 takes the form of a question: is there midbrain above the level of cranial nerve (CN) III complex? (Answer:

yes.) The question invites another: what's above the midbrain? Which leads to yet one more: what's the boundary between midbrain (also known as mesencephalon) and the diencephalon immediately above and contiguous with it?

*

> **RULE #4**: More a convention than a rule, we'll apply the following to all our axial sections: ventral brainstem is *below* dorsal brainstem. (If you look at MR or CT images of brain, ventral brainstem is *above* dorsal brainstem.)

THE DI-MESENCEPHALON. The diencephalon, as we recall from developmental anatomy (so long ago, for me), consists of four strata best visualized early in embryonic life: from dorsal to ventral, they are the *epithalamus* (destined to become the pineal gland and habenular nuclei, among other things), *dorsal thalamus* (which will develop into thalamus and all its nuclei), *subthalamus* ("a continuation of the midbrain tegmentum"), and *hypothalamus* (Kahle, 1986). So, honestly, is there a clear division between midbrain/mesencephalon and diencephalon, if the midbrain tegmentum continues into subthalamus, among whose structures is the subthalamic nucleus of Luys?

I'm obsessing about the border for two reasons. First, the di-mesencephalic boundary is discrete, based on gene expression in development: PAX6 is found in telencephalon and diencephalon down to the di-mesencephalic boundary, at which border (only after crossing it, heading inferiorly) there's expression of genes like En1, En2, and PAX 2 (Nakamura, 2001). All the above genes are implicated in the differentiation (the regionalization) of mesencephalon as opposed to prosencephalon–the latter includes both diencephalon and telencephalon. Increasingly, anatomy isn't just dissection and photomicrography anymore, since genes govern anatomic relations. Second, if you happen to consult good neuroanatomy atlases (e.g., DeArmond et al., 1989), you can't help but notice that *oblique axial sections result in images in which structures at different vertical levels appear in the same picture.* For example, thalamic nuclei can show up in axial sections of the most rostral midbrain, given the vertical proximity of thalamus (and other diencephalic structures) and the mesencephalon. All of thalamus is diencephalic, and the midbrain is mesencephalic–which is to say, they're different, but they're neighbors. The same can be said of hypothalamus and mesencephalon.

Imagine a midbrain section *above* the level of CN III nuclear complex, and you'll visualize both the **red nuclei** and two other round nuclear structures dorsal to the red nuclei—all four are close to the midline. The dorsal ones must be thalamic; you're visualizing the circular centromedian nuclei of thalamus which are dorsal and superior to the red nuclei. If you're not familiar with any thalamic nuclei, then perhaps there's incentive for me to write a monograph about them. But the point is not to be confused or befuddled if presented with a non-canonical image of midbrain. (By canonical in this context, I refer to a midbrain image in which we clearly see the midline, shark's-tooth, or V-shaped appearance of cranial nerve III complex, about which more later).

At the di-mesencephalic transition, you might visualize a wispy white-matter tract crossing the axial midline from side to side. We're not referring to the monstrously large *corpus callosum* connecting *hemispheres* with each other. At the current, very rostral level of *midbrain*—above the level of the superior colliculi—there are really only two options as to what the thing is: the habenular commissure or the posterior commissure, both of epithalamic origin. The posterior commissure is much larger than the other. But the thin **habenular commissure** is interesting, because you might notice that there's a bit of gland (not white matter) in the midline, just dorsal to it. That's the pineal gland, which is epithalamic/diencephalic, not mesencephalic.

The rostral, dorsal mesencephalon, which we're discussing and which derives from a dorsal (or alar) plate, differentiates into an **optic tectum**, a term most familiar to vertebrate neuroanatomists (Sato et al., 2004). The optic tectum has cellular lamination similar to that seen in visual neocortex, and the optic tectum is a terminus of optic tract in many animals, but not in humans (Carpenter and Sutin, 1983). In other words, you could envision the very rostral midbrain and the superior colliculus, which we're about to introduce, as preeminently and phylogenetically *sensory and visual*.

I haven't discussed the ventral bulk of midbrain at this level (people refer to a midbrain tegmentum, but the etymology confuses me; as in the word integument, the root of *tegmentum* refers to a cover; anatomists talk about how the brainstem covers the ventricular system, but I think it's an odd term nevertheless). **Red nucleus** resides in midbrain tegmentum; ventral to red nucleus, there's also *substantia nigra*; dorsolateral to the *substantia nigra* is the lens-shaped **subthalamic nucleus of Luys,** which is of diencephalic origin (it derives from the stratum called subthalamus).

There are the fiber tracts which connect globus pallidus and thalamus via the upper midbrain, including an ***ansa lenticularis*** (*ansa*, Latin = loop) and a **lenticular fasciculus**. The *ansa lenticularis* and lenticular fasciculus will converge into the **thalamic fasciculus,** one of whose destinations is the ***zona incerta,*** a ventral continuation of the reticular nucleus of thalamus (Haubenberger and Hallett, 2018 describe the significance of the above anatomy to tremor). All the fiber tracts just mentioned illustrate how midbrain continues into subthalamus and thalamus.

Note to self: there are surgical interventions for the treatment of tremor that target the *zona incerta* of thalamus. If a lesion is placed, for example, in or near the left *zona incerta*, a reduction in tremor will manifest in the contralateral (right) hemibody. If somebody didn't have a tremor, but suffered a stroke in left *zona incerta*, would tremor result? Dunno, but, if a tremor appeared, it would be contralateral to the side of the lesion.

I haven't discussed the bulk of midbrain at this level, because I'm waiting for the first evidence of the **quadrigeminal plate** and, in association with it, the posterior commissure.

30

Just at the Superior Colliculi

Let's move just a bit inferiorly, to the rostral border of the superior colliculi. Nieuwenhuys et al. (2008) cite the dorsal, ventral, and lateral boundaries of our new axial section:

> The border of the mesencephalon with the diencephalon is set caudal to the *posterior commissure* dorsally and caudal to the *mamillary bodies* ventrally. . . . Laterally, it [the midbrain] follows the caudal border of the optic tracts, where the pes pedunculi emerges on the ventral surface. The geniculate bodies and the pulvinar of the thalamus are located lateral to the rostral mesencephalon.

Despite its textbook authority, the description disorients me. Didn't we just say that the posterior commissure is epithalamic in origin–i.e., above the midbrain? The mamillary bodies belong to posterior hypothalamus, also diencephalic. It won't suffice to say that diencephalon and mesencephalon live on discrete floors of a building. It's not that simple.

Try a thought experiment. Think about a cone. Invert it (apex or vertex pointing down), as if you held an empty ice-cream (sugar) cone. Now imagine an oblique conic section that creates an ellipse rather than a neat circle at the top. We're interested only in the upper/dorsal part of the ellipse–the location, in other words, of the rostral tips of the two **superior**

colliculi and a **pretectal area** (before, ventral, and superior to superior colliculus).

The largest transverse white matter tract that you see at this level is the posterior commissure, which appears very early in the developing human brain, at about ten weeks' gestational age.

The cone in our hand is a three-dimensional shape. What's around it neuroanatomically?

Answers, in terms of anatomic relationships, at the level of the uppermost midbrain:

> VENTRALLY: actually, NOTHING except the cerebrospinal fluid of the interpeduncular fossa (the space between either crus cerebri or cerebral peduncle or pes pedunculi). The mamillary bodies of hypothalamus are also located in that interpeduncular fossa.

> DORSALLY: actually, NOTHING, except for the cerebrospinal fluid of the quadrigeminal plate cistern.

> LATERALLY: The answer *depends*. Dorsolaterally, there are grey structures symmetrically on either side, because thalamic nuclei (especially, the medial and lateral geniculate bodies) drape over the sides of the midbrain . . . only dorsolaterally. Ventrolaterally, optic tracts wrap themselves around the cerebral peduncles on either side.

Note the physical proximity of these structures, which we've identified so far:

> **posterior commissure;**
> **pretectal area;**
> **superior colliculi** (homologous to the vertebrate optic tectum);
> **optic tracts;** and
> thalamic nuclei, in particular, the **lateral geniculate bodies.**

In experiments dating to the 1930's, stimulation of posterior commissure, pretectal area, superior colliculus, optic tract, and areas near but not in the lateral geniculate bodies all produced bilateral pupillary constriction. One might think that either an isolated pretectal lesion or a precise lesion in posterior commissure should disrupt a consensual light reflex, but it appears that only major midbrain damage in pretectal area and posterior commissure *together* impairs expected bilateral pupillary constriction when light is presented to one eye (Carpenter and Pierson, 1973).

We haven't reached an axial section that includes any obvious cranial nerve nucleus, yet we have already discussed much about eyes. We teach that the direct and consensual light response is a reflex whose connections are mesencephalic (optic tract to pretectal area to posterior commissure, without cortical connections).

By comparison, we say that accommodation, otherwise known as the near reflex, involves projections to and from visual cortex. The projection *from* cortex goes *to* midbrain—but where in midbrain? Answer: very high in it, perhaps specifically in rostral superior colliculus in both accommodation and active fixation (Ohtsuka and Nagasaka, 1999).

We talk about saccade generation originating in frontal cortex, in the frontal eye fields, but how often do we think about how the rostral mesencephalon, especially the superior colliculi, might be responsible for getting eyes to look at certain targets and not others? Hikosaka et al. (2000) beautifully discuss that visual (and maybe not just visual) maps of the world converge in the superior colliculi, and that visual search and saccades were functions that emerged in evolution with the establishment of cortico-superior collicular connections.

In discussing eyes in all five instances (light reflex, accommodation, active fixation, saccade generation, visual scanning), the rostral mesencephalon is like a funnel through which many visual pathways necessarily pass.

*

POSTERIOR COMMISSURE AND THE UPPER AQUEDUCT OF SYLVIUS (CEREBRAL AQUEDUCT). In the upper middle of midbrain at this level sits the cerebral aqueduct, ventral to posterior commissure. Grey matter (**periaqueductal grey**) surrounds the sides of the aqueduct. Once I see the posterior commissure, I know the cerebral aqueduct is ventral to it. Period.

The opposite is not true: if you see the cerebral aqueduct, it doesn't mean that the posterior commissure is necessarily above it. At other levels, the periaqueductal grey completely surrounds the aqueduct.

We're now in a position to organize our thinking about the midbrain in general. I think of the midpoint of the cerebral aqueduct in midbrain and rostral pons as part of a side-to-side border between up/dorsal and down/ventral in brainstem.

I'm oversimplifying. There's debate over whether a division between basal and alar plates exists as high as the midbrain (Mastick and Easter, 1996). Lower in the brainstem, particularly in the medulla, we can point to a sulcus (described by Wilhelm His, Sr.) that divides alar and basal plates, but no such landmark exists in midbrain. Yet we can roughly group nuclei above/dorsal and below/ventral to aqueduct in midbrain.

We divide into alar/dorsal and basal/ventral based on sensory and motor nuclei, *respectively.* If we think about the ventral or dorsal location of white-matter tracts or of cranial-nerve fascicles, we'll get confused, especially further down in the brainstem. Alar/dorsal *nuclei* are sensory; basal/ventral *nuclei* are motoric. I can't call it a law; it's just a serviceable principle.

DORSAL/ALAR/SENSORY NUCLEI. Above/dorsal to the cerebral aqueduct, we have the superior colliculi.

*

But what's to be said about these structures, from medial to lateral, on both sides of periaqueductal grey, *just at the level* of the aqueduct:

> **nucleus of Darkschewitsch** and
> **interstitial nucleus of Cajal.**

We'll add:

> **rostral-interstitial nucleus of the medial longitudinal fasciculus (MLF).**

All three are close to each other and to the MLF (yes, MLF is present above the level of CN III nuclei); all structures abut the periaqueductal grey on either side.

Fibers arising from all three nuclei enter the posterior commissure. All three nuclei are, in some sense, sensory, insofar as they receive vestibulocerebellar input and somatosensory information about the position of the head and neck in space. But no anatomist would comfortably call the nuclei of Darkschewitsch, interstitial nuclei of Cajal, and rostral-interstitial nuclei of MLF purely sensory, given the pre-motor or accessory oculomotor role of all three in the control of eye movements (for a representative discussion, see Fukushima, 1987).

I'll abide by my organizing principle: dorsal to the posterior commissure and to the cerebral aqueduct are the **superior colliculi (optic tectum)**. Those are sensory nuclei just as the lateral geniculate body of thalamus is a sensory nucleus. In fact, the superior colliculi are multisensory, because they integrate more than visual afferent information. Stimulate a right superior colliculus: eyes (conjugately), head, and neck turn to the left. Nauta and Feirtag (1986) talk about how, late at night, if you heard a mosquito, your head orients/turns in the direction of the buzzing intruder: the (multisensory) superior colliculus is involved even in that darkness.

*

Lateral to the cerebral aqueduct, we encounter white-matter tracts:

> **central tegmental tract** (a visible portion of the reticular formation, about which we will have a bit to say, but not now),

> **spinothalamic, and medial lemniscal tracts**.

Very laterally, we're already outside of mesencephalon, because we see medial and lateral geniculate bodies of thalamus.

VENTRAL/BASAL/MOTOR NUCLEI. We see **red nucleus**– "red," because in fresh brain dissections, it looks pink, which is to say iron-reddish. Then there are motor tracts ventral to red nucleus, specifically the three portions of the (ventral) crus cerebri or cerebral peduncle, including, medial to lateral: a **frontopontine tract**, so-called Arnold's bundle, heading inferiorly to pontine nuclei; a central third of the crus which contains corticospinal fibers, many of which will form the pyramid in medulla; and a lateral third of the crus which contains a **temporopontine tract**, so-called Türck's bundle, also headed to pontine nuclei.

The hard-to-miss red nucleus is a defining ventral motor nucleus of the rostral mesencephalon.

The **rubrospinal tract** arises from it, but it's also the terminus of some fibers from contralateral deep cerebellar nuclei.

Ventral to red nucleus, but dorsal to the crus cerebri (its three parts), are the *pars compacta* and *pars reticulata* of the *substantia nigra*. At the level we now discuss, we're below the subthalamic nucleus of Luys, which is no longer visible.

The black, neuromelanin-containing cells of the *pars compacta* differ from neurons in *the pars reticulata*. Reticular neurons behave physiologically like pallidal neurons in the globus pallidus *pars interna*. *Compacta* neurons are dopaminergic, related to a nigrostriatal pathway that will pass into a **median forebrain bundle** (also known as the medial telencephalic fascicle) medial to the **central tegmental tract**, which we identified previously, en route to the *corpus striatum* (Moore and Bloom, 1978).

I'd draw attention to the often overlooked, *other* dopaminergic **ventral tegmental area of Tsai**, which is dorsomedial to both parts of *substantia nigra* and ventral to red nucleus in the interpeduncular midline. Its axons, also via **medial forebrain bundle**, project widely to prefrontal cortex (for an introductory discussion, see Goldman-Rakic, 1999).

Note to self: red nucleus on one side deals with contralateral hemibody (a left lesion results in right-sided findings in the body). Why? By the time you see the (left) red nucleus, cerebellar fibers have already crossed from (right) contralateral deep cerebellar nuclei. But: most axons from the *pars compacta* of the *substantia nigra* project to *ipsilateral corpus striatum* via the homolateral median forebrain bundle. The *pars compacta* is an extrapyramidal, motoric nucleus. Also: ventral tegmental area projects to ipsilateral cortex (Coenen et al., 2018). Learning which tracts cross the midline and which ones don't causes pain for students universally, I know. As discussed in the first seminar, the organization of the brain isn't always crossed.

Cortico-ponto-cerebellar projections (the bundles of Arnold [medial] and Türck [lateral]) reside on either side of pyramidal-tract fibers in the cerebral peduncle. The **red nucleus** hovers dorsal to the cerebral peduncle.

Could an acute, unilateral lesion at this level result in a combination of ataxia and hemiparesis in the contralateral hemibody? If you think so, then how do you to explain the *isolated* foot drop in the case from chapter 28?

31

At the Levels of CN III Complex

The plural is intentional: it's a simple fact that the large CN III complex occupies midline vertical space from the moment we visualize it through all axial sections down to the CN IV nucleus, which has been described as "a small caudal appendage of the oculomotor nuclear complex" (Carpenter and Sutin, 1983).

*

> **RULE #5**. Find the cerebral aqueduct. If you don't find
> it, you're not in midbrain.

Please don't misread the rule. There's cerebral aqueduct in the rostral pons as well. The rule only says that there's cerebral aqueduct in midbrain. If you see fourth ventricle, you're not in midbrain.

*

DORSAL/ALAR/SENSORY NUCLEI. Having applied **RULE #5**, I notice that there's periaqueductal grey all around the aqueduct, but there's no posterior commissure, because we're now below it.

I apply the principle that nuclei dorsal to/above the level of the aqueduct are sensory. Aside from the **superior colliculus**, there's only one other sensory nucleus of note, the **mesencephalic nucleus of CN V**, located along the lateral edge of the periaqueductal grey. It's curious for being a dorsal root ganglion inside brainstem parenchyma. Fibers arrive there by way a mesencephalic tract of CN V; its afferent information relates to proprioception of the teeth and "the force of the bite" (Carpenter and Sutin, 1983).

VENTRAL/BASAL/MOTOR NUCLEI. We'll concentrate on CN III complex, but we first re-acknowledge white matter tracts that we encountered in the previous axial section, all lateral to red nucleus:

> **central tegmental tract** (a visible portion of the reticular formation, superior to the red nucleus),
> and, laterally,
> the **spinothalamic and medial lemniscal tracts.**

Very (dorso)laterally, we're already outside of mesencephalon, because we see medial geniculate body of thalamus; lateral geniculate body has passed out of our field of view.

*

Oculomotor nucleus (we'll discuss just one side of CN III nuclear complex) resides beneath/ventral to the cerebral aqueduct at the ventral margin of the periaqueductal grey. It contains motor neurons that innervate the following muscles:

> medial rectus (MR)
> inferior rectus (IR)
> *contralateral* superior rectus (*contralateral* SR)
> inferior oblique (IO)
> *levator palpebrae* (LP)

In addition, the parasympathetic Edinger-Westphal nucleus sends preganglionic fibers that synapse at the ciliary ganglion in the orbit: it's involved not only in the control of pupillary constriction (via action of the pupillary sphincter), but also accommodation and blood flow to the ciliary muscle (the latter responsible for changing the shape of the lens in the near reflex). There's both a preganglionic Edinger-Westphal nucleus and a centrally projecting Edinger Westphal nucleus–the latter contains a neuropeptide transmitter called urocortin; its central projections aren't entirely clear–perhaps to hypothalamus, the serotonergic dorsal raphe, and even spinal cord (May et al., 2008).

The CN III nuclear complex has subnuclei that are discrete in the vertical space (the ensuing discussion follows Ngwa et al., 2014). There's value in knowing about the location of subnuclei, because you improve your understanding about eye movements in both the vertical and horizontal planes.

*

MR subnucleus first. Just a moment ago, we created a list; there's an intentional and anatomical order to it, from rostral to caudal:

MR, IR, contralateral SR, IO, LP.

Begin, rostrally, with MR subnucleus. Actually, MR subnucleus in humans is present at all axial levels of CN III complex; there are subdivisions of MR subnucleus. But along with the Edinger-Westphal nucleus, at the most rostral extent of the CN III complex *is* a MR subnucleus. Why does this high location make sense?

We've alluded to accommodation or the near reflex, and at very least we know that in accommodating, both eyes adduct at the same time. We've mentioned that rostral superior colliculus or perhaps the pretectal area (what some people call a supraoculomotor area) may be involved in the cortically mediated act of accommodation. A powerful, excitatory vergence input gets both eyes to adduct; we must assume that there's concurrent decrease in firing of the muscle yoked to MR–i.e., a decrease in firing rate of lateral rectus, a muscle we haven't discussed yet (Büttner-Ennever, 2006). MR subnucleus is rostral, as are locales that mediate the brainstem pathways involved in accommodation.

There's an issue, however. The Edinger-Westphal sub-nucleus at this very rostral level contains urocortin (centrally projecting), and is not strictly pre-ganglionic/parasympathetic. The clearest visualization of parasympathetic Edinger-Westphal nucleus happens some millimeters below where we are (at which level we see all CN III extraocular subnuclei together, in the canonical section which depicts CN III's shark's tooth shape). But preganglionic Edinger-Westphal neurons are diffusely present in the midline CN III complex, even when we can't point to the parasympathetic subnucleus itself.

*

MR and IR subnuclei together. The next subnucleus we encounter is IR. When we see MR and IR subnuclei together, anatomists also identify an unpaired, midline nucleus Perlia (it's yet another CN III subnucleus; Richard Perlia described it in 1889). Nucleus Perlia was once thought to be involved in convergence, but later studies haven't confirmed that hypothesis. These days, some people think that it's involved in upgaze.

MR and IR subnuclei are present together in all subsequent caudal sections.

A primary action of IR in the vertical plane is depression of the eye, especially but not only in abduction. But when I think about the near reflex (or if I just look at my own nose, crossing and depressing my eyes to do so), I intuit that the anatomical proximity of MR and IR subnuclei makes sense. Someone will ask about the role of superior oblique, but we haven't arrived at its nucleus yet. (In any event, looking straight down involves *both* IR and superior oblique muscles.)

MR, IR, IO, and *contralateral* SR subnuclei together. At the next caudal level, all CN III subnuclei involved in control of its associated extraocular muscles are present in one axial section.

We've discussed the grouping of IR/IO/contralateral SR in the first seminar. It's vain, but I'll cut and paste what I wrote; the subject matter is what happens in both eyes when a quick, vertical corrective saccade happens:

> . . . in a run we take one random day, with one footfall, there's a pothole we didn't expect. It's an irregular pothole. A foot gets caught in an oblique way, casting us in an oblique downward direction, but, mercifully, we don't fall. The run continues to our satisfaction, without injury.
>
> As foot meets pothole, I envision events having occurred within just a few milliseconds: unilateral firing of the rostral interstitial nucleus of the MLF, say, on the left, then immediate activation of the following, all on the

same side of the midline (on the left): subnuclei of inferior oblique, inferior rectus, [contralateral] superior rectus, *and* the left trochlear nucleus [which innervates contralateral superior oblique]. The result, with short latency between nuclear discharge and muscle action involving the eyes: a corrective saccade involving the left inferior oblique and inferior rectus acting on the left eye, and an equal saccade of contralateral superior rectus and the superior oblique acting on the right eye.

There's sense in the grouping of IR, IO, and *contralateral* SR subnuclei.

The central caudal nucleus. The most caudal of the CN III subnuclei is an unpaired nucleus which contains motor neurons that innervate the *levator palpebrae* on either side. It's not clear why, but motor neurons in the central caudate nucleus are mainly inhibited by GABA-ergic neurons located at the level of the posterior commissure.

Imagine a combination of findings, as Henri Parinaud introduced them in 1883: a main finding is an upgaze paresis in both eyes; the paresis could be bad enough that the eyes look downward in the primary position ("sun setting" eyes); in attempting upgaze, the eyelid widens so that you see a good bit of white sclera above the limbus of the iris (Collier's sign, a failure in normal inhibition of central caudal nucleus); also in attempting upgaze, sometimes there's a nystagmus in which the fast phase moves towards the midline in both eyes, a convergence nystagmus; yet accommodation is poor (in fact, the pupils look dilated, and they stay that way). People refer to a syndrome of the cerebral aqueduct; it's a good term, because multiple levels of CN III complex must be involved to produce its constellation of signs.

32

They Stare at Me

In my first year teaching neuroanatomy, I regularly identified the CN IV (trochlear) nuclei as part of the midline structure called CN III nucleus. I made the mistake consistently. Since then, I've been fascinated by young teachers' errors (and those of old academics, too; I still err often). The missteps are unintentional, of course. Yet I still wonder whether an innocent lapse points to some confusion inherent in our nomenclature or in our understanding. The medial lemniscus isn't the medial longitudinal fasciculus, for example. The median forebrain bundle isn't found only in the forebrain. A subtler error, still related to a problem with names, is a confusion between a/the nucleus/i of the posterior commissure (there are such nuclei) and, say, the interstitial nucleus of Cajal and the nucleus of Darkschewitsch, both of whose fibers project into posterior commissure. Is a phenomenon like Collier's sign, mentioned at the end of the last chapter, the result of a nuclear lesion or of a white-matter disconnection of some type? A last example among so many accrued over years would be the thought that one can't distinguish the inferior from superior colliculus in a random axial section. Wrong. One can. The superior one is laminated; the inferior one isn't.

Let's state the obvious for the record: nobody at any school or anywhere else seeks embarrassment by way of their misstatements, but they're universal and common—both the misstatements and the embarrassment.

A cover-up that often ensues is usually far worse than the error was in the first place.

It's all perfectly OK; we're just trying to learn.

*

All the same, as I think about an axial section of midbrain below the level of the central caudal nucleus, I see in front of my eyes the bright, beacon-like, neatly round, small, midline-hugging CN IV nuclei. They stare at me, and they're all the more obvious when the section is stained such that white matter is black. Blackness of white matter in a Weil or Loyez stain makes CN IV nuclei even more obvious in their intimate relationship to the very dark medial longitudinal fasciculus (MLF), in which the nuclei are nestled. We know that MLF exists above the level of CN III nuclear complex, and we'll see how it extends well below CN VI nuclei in the pons.

Assuming that one doesn't have a demonic axial section that cuts very obliquely, the colliculus at the level of CN IV nuclei is inferior, not superior.

We apply our principle related to the cerebral aqueduct in midbrain and rostral pons. Per **RULE #5** (find the cerebral aqueduct; if you don't find it, you're not in midbrain), it's there, surrounded by periaqueductal grey, so midbrain is a reasonable, albeit not exclusive possibility regarding our location (remember, cerebral aqueduct is also present in the high pons).

Now we divide and organize.

DORSAL/ALAR/SENSORY NUCLEI. We'll concentrate on **inferior colliculus**, the conspicuous sensory nucleus in our current field of view. Yet we should re-acknowledge the presence, at this level as in the last, of the mesencephalic nucleus of CN V in the lateral borders of the periaqueductal grey on either side.

*

The inferior colliculus contributes to an attention to sound rather than to physical characteristics like sound frequency, intensity, interaural time differences between either ear, etc. (Ono and Ito, 1985). I like the phrase "attention to sound." It evokes the sense of a head turn towards an unseen target as a function of superior colliculus. Both the superior and inferior colliculi are somewhat mis-described as being visual and auditory, respectively, because there are ways in which both structures must be multimodal.

Regarding inferior colliculus, I have an idiosyncratic view of it. So, here's a vignette and digression.

I use my 128-hertz tuning fork everyday to test patients' vibratory sense (the lemniscal pathway). I strike the fork; I apply it to the great toe. Over the years, I've come to tap the fork ever so lightly. In medical school, I banged it like *Homo habilis* with an early tool in fist. Then as now, obviously, I'm producing sound waves of different intensities, but my intention with my 128-hertz instrument at someone's foot is to test a system that starts with a mechanoreceptor in soft tissue, not to test hearing. The sensory pathway I test shares the word lemniscus with a structure in the auditory pathway. (The *medial* lemniscus relates to how vibratory information finds its way to somatosensory thalamus; the *lateral* lemniscus has to do with the auditory pathway. A lemniscus is a ribbon-like structure, and indeed both medial and lateral lemnisci ribbon-wind their way rostrally.)

It should come as no surprise that the **lateral lemniscus** is present in our current axial section; its white matter seems part of the inferior colliculi. The lateral lemniscus is dorsal to both the medial lemniscus and the spinothalamic tract. The lateral lemniscus differs from yet another tract that's also quite lateral in midbrain, the **brachium of inferior colliculus**. The latter is lateral to *both* the inferior and superior colliculi in consecutive axial sections. The *brachium* of inferior colliculus connects inferior colliculus to medial geniculate body of thalamus. It's not a direct continuation of lateral lemniscus.

Memories have a peculiar way of sticking together. When I used to bang at my turning fork, my patients regularly said, "yes, I hear that." How could they not? Then, in a separate but related memory, for years upon years, I watched colleagues and students point in the general area of the lateral, dorsal midbrain, and they'd say "there's medial lemniscus, or *brachium* of inferior colliculus, or lateral lemniscus, or spinothalamic tract. *They're all there.*" Those persons weren't incorrect; but it all seemed hand-wavingly vague to me. But my glued-together memories have left me with a notion that there must be relationship between auditory and tactile vibrations.

Enter the interesting question (to me) of whether snakes—boas, rattlesnakes, what have you—*hear*, or whether they primarily sense ground vibration. As it happens, the structures of the snake jaw—a columella akin to stapes; a quadrate akin to incus; and the snake mandible, which contacts the ground as malleus contacts the tympanic membrane—serve as inner-ear ossicles. And, just to let you know, snakes have eighth cranial nerves.

The supposedly earless snake. hears both by sound and by ground vibration, and *both data sets project onto a snake's version of the inferior colliculus* (Hartline, 1971). I think about that observation whenever I see inferior colliculus, and—I whisper this next part to myself—maybe there's a reason for the anatomical proximity of a facial proprioceptive center (mesencephalic nucleus of CN V, related to the jaw, no less) and the fiber tracts of the medial and lateral lemnisci.

*

VENTRAL/BASAL/MOTOR NUCLEI. Here's an official-sounding description of **CN IV nucleus**: "The trochlear nucleus (IV) lies in the midbrain ventral to the aquaeduct [sic]. In humans, it has been observed to consist of one large [motor neuron or 'motoneuron'] group 'sunken' into the MLF; and several smaller groups of motoneurons further caudally. . . .. It contains only motoneurons of the contralateral superior oblique [SO] muscle; however the contribution of SO motor unit activity during some types of eye movements such as convergence . . . is still not well understood" (Büttner-Ennever, 2006). I quote the passage for two reasons.

The first has to do with an idea, mentioned at the start of the last chapter and the beginning of this one, that CN IV nucleus represents a caudal appendage of CN III nuclear complex. If little motoneuron collections extend further caudally from the more-obvious, central bulk of CN IV nucleus, then couldn't we start to envision a very medially located column of somatic motoneurons beginning in midbrain?

One approach to brainstem has been to organize it into functional units that span the rostral-caudal axis, though "the classical division of the brainstem into *functional columns* has been a problem because it has proved difficult to delimit terms . . ." (my italics, Müller and O'Rahilly, 2011). I agree: terms like special vs. general visceral efferent don't help me as much as they might other people. We'll address columns when we arrive in medulla.

Second, the author doesn't say that CN IV nucleus *uniquely* innervates a contralateral muscle, because we know of other subnuclei that involve either complete or partial decussation to their respective muscles–e.g., the superior rectus subnucleus or the central caudal nucleus, as discussed in the last chapter.

Nevertheless, since CN IV motoneurons innervate contralateral superior oblique motor units, then the infranuclear fascicle or the nerve itself must cross the midline. The former claim about the fascicle, not the latter about the extra-axial nerve, is true: "Root [fascicular] fibers emerging from the [CN IV] nucleus curve dorsolaterally and caudally in the outer margin of the central [periaqueductal] gray, decussate completely in the superior medullary velum and exit from the dorsal surface of the brain stem caudal to the inferior colliculus" (Carpenter and Sutin, 1983).

*

We've concentrated on CN IV nuclei, but we should re-acknowledge the white matter tracts we've previously encountered:

> **central tegmental tract** (a still-visible portion of the reticular formation, lateral to a centrally located decussation of the superior cerebellar peduncles; the red nuclei are no longer visible, because we are below them),
> and, laterally,
> the **spinothalamic and medial lemniscal tracts**.

We're not done with **VENTRAL/MOTOR NUCLEI** aside from CN IV nuclei. But on the subject of white matter tracts ventral to the inferior colliculi, one must ask, with amazement, if not incredulity: why all the white-matter midline crossings at our present axial level?

In the 1940's, an anatomist wondered whether the trochlear decussation had to do with the embryonic appearance of the cerebellum (Cooper, 1947). At the level of the inferior colliculi, the dominant decussation we see is that of the superior cerebellar peduncles (in an appropriately stained section, it's a big blob of black inside the midline tegmentum, dorsal to the cerebral peduncles), but there are other crossings worth considering. At the isthmus between lower midbrain and the remaining hindbrain a number of transactions happen in limited anatomic space:

deep cerebellar nuclear axons (they ascend) cross to the contralateral red nuclei (as mentioned, via the **decussation of the superior cerebellar peduncles** or *brachia conjunctivae*);

tectum (particularly, the superior colliculus) projects to spinal cord (the projections descend and cross in the **dorsal tegmental decussation**, which is also known as **the fountain decussation of Meynert**);

tectum projects to mesencephalic reticular formation (bilaterally) and to contralateral pontine and medullary reticular formation (also via the dorsal tegmental decussation);

and red nucleus projects either to contralateral spinal cord (the projections descend and cross in the **ventral tegmental decussation**), or they project to ipsilateral medulla, without decussation, via the **central tegmental tract** (Nathan and Smith, 1982).

So, at the level of the trochlear decussation and the decussation of the superior cerebellar peduncles, we pivot to the bridge that is pons:

The decussation of the trochlear nerve in the superior medullary velum and the rostral edge of the pons mark the border of the mesencephalon [read: midbrain] and the metencephalon [read: pons] on the dorsal and ventral sides of the brainstem, respectively, and the decussation of the superior cerebellar peduncle marks the transition of the tegmentum pontis into the tegmentum mescenphali (Nieuwenhuys et al., 2008).

In some sections of low midbrain, you visualize the transition from cerebral peduncles to the tegmentum pontis. And in that ventral domain are **VENTRAL/MOTOR NUCLEI** in abundance, specifically the pontine nuclei, about which more when we get to pons.

*

RULE #6. The person who says it's not important clinically could be horribly mistaken.

RULE #6 is just an opinion based on many hours watching how we teach students. Out of necessity, we choose certain things to emphasize—that's both proper and practical. But throwing out too many details is like dismissing pertinent positives in talking with patients. The consequences of doing so can be less than delightful.

So, what's a person to do? One can't commit everything to memory.

Here's an approach that I've found useful, if time consuming. Based on curiosity alone, ask "what *is* that?" Then, if you're so inclined, you spend hours ferreting out your answer. I have two examples in mind, as we prepare to depart from midbrain to pons.

Example 1: the periaqueductal (or central) grey. It's grey or (if you prefer the occidental spelling) gray, right? So, it must consist of neurons, but are they divisible into dorsal/sensory and ventral/motor populations? We admitted from the start that our alar/basal dividing line in midbrain and rostral pons is an oversimplification. Moreno-Bravo et al. (2012) note that genetic differentiation to distinguish alar or basal plate neuronal origin in the periaqueductal grey is less well characterized than elsewhere in the midbrain, but they also note that although there are neurons there, they don't obviously collect into nuclei.

But we continue to ask: what *is* it? Nauta and Feirtag (1986) teach about the periaqueductal grey effortlessly; the italics are mine:

> The central gray substance has long been known as a destination for fibers that travel with the spinothalamic tract *but do not attain the thalamus*. It also receives projections from cerebral cortex, the hypothalamus, and the reticular formation. Its outputs are no less heterogeneous: it projects upward to the hypothalamus and the superior colliculus, *radially outward to the surrounding reticular formation, and downward to the rhombencephalic reticular formation*, the nucleus of the solitary tract, and the dorsal motor nucleus of the vagus.

The only part of the surrounding mesencephalic reticular formation that we've visualized is the central tegmental tract, which passes from red nucleus to caudal points (it also contains fibers which ascend to cortex). But there's a larger network/reticulum that we don't see, though it's invisibly present, as someone once described *the* nothing that is, throughout the brainstem.

Example 2: *I'll withhold the name for a moment.* Between exiting fascicles of both oculomotor nerves, in the very ventral tegmentum, *immediately* dorsal to the interpeduncular fossa, is a midline, solitary nucleus that's close to the ventral tegmental area of Tsai. It has pigmented cells in it. What *is* that?

(Trust me: the more you ask the question sincerely, the more you learn. For a discussion of the connectivities we invoke by identifying this structure, see Hikosaka, 2010.)

Its name describes its location: the **interpeduncular nucleus**, which is highly conserved across vertebrate species. It communicates with epithalamus via *fasciculus retroflexus* or the **habenula-interpeduncular tract**, whose medially placed fibers contribute to what seems like a white-matter capsule surrounding the red nuclei on either side. Recall that we started at the interface between epithalamus and mesencephalon. Here, as we leave midbrain, there's a structure in bent-back communication with rostral epithalamus. It's not a somatic motor nucleus; it *is* of basal plate origin; it receives from the habenulae, and it projects to midline nuclei in the raphe, a seam or suture (from the Greek), best seen in pons.

33

Rostral Pons

The look of the cerebral aqueduct has changed. In midbrain, it's more or less a circle. At the transition to the pons, I'd say that it looks quadrilateral. The dorsal two edges, which meet in the midline to form an inverted letter V, form the thin roof which we identified in the previous chapter as the **superior medullary velum**. Infranuclear fascicles from CN IV nuclei decussate through it. (Depending on the brain you're studying, the circular aqueduct could also change its appearance to something more like a Y shape; the point's still the same: it's look has changed.) We're at the rostral extent of the fourth ventricle, but atlases still refer to the cerebral aqueduct's presence in the high pons.

Applying the principle that **DORSAL/ALAR/SENSORY NUCLEI** lie above the aqueduct, we find mesencephalic nucleus of CN V on either side of the aqueduct, dorsal to a bluish nucleus which appears at this level.

The superior medullary velum is of alar-plate origin as the cerebellum is of alar-plate origin. So, one can't say that alar structures have vanished; rather, the superior medullary velum is a first suggestion of cerebellum (Müller and O'Rahilly, 1988). As an aside, both the pons and the cerebellar hemispheres in humans are inordinately large compared to all other species.

Superior, middle, and inferior cerebellar peduncles–the three white-matter struts which connect brainstem to cerebellum and vice versa–will serve as landmarks for the remainder of our tour.

*

To clarify terms, there are people who refer to the dorsal/upper half of the pons at this level as the **pontine tegmentum**, whereas the ventral/lower/larger portion goes by names like the pons proper or the *basis pontis*. (Note the difference, compared to midbrain: tectum is dorsal and tegmentum is ventral.) There's still a roof (tectum) in the rostral pons, however: the **superior medullary velum**, and, more caudally, the **inferior medullary velum** cover the fourth ventricle, which widens as we pass lower into the pons, are both alar and tectal. Structures like the superior cerebellar peduncle, the extensive white matter of the middle cerebellar peduncle, the inferior cerebellar peduncle, and cerebellum itself will also dorsally tent the fourth ventricle. More on all those structures in time.

The 16th century Italian anatomist, Constanzo Varolio, who first assigned the term "pons" to pons, thought that it was a bridge (in Italian, *ponte*; in French, *pont*; in Latin, *pons*) between cerebellar hemispheres. His 1573 book contains a curious illustration in which he split the brainstem lengthwise while it's still attached to the brain, then he splayed the brainstem's two lengthwise halves in different directions; he had to have cut the dorsal midline cerebellum to accomplish this perspective (Bahsi et al., 2018). Varolio thought that pons was a passage from side to side, not from hemispheres to hindbrain.

In axial section, the *basis pontis* to me looks symmetrical from side to side just as the midbrain does, but instead of ventral cerebral peduncles, we have the appearance of a slightly cleft chin (a large one, a bit bilobed) with a midline seam or suture that passes from the ventral surface all the way to the cerebral aqueduct. If you visualize the great amount of white matter in the *basis pontis*, some fibers seem pass from side to side and others pass from above to below.

In the tegmentum ventral to the aqueduct, we re-acknowledge the white matter tracts we've previously encountered:

> **medial longitudinal fasciculus** at the midline, ventral to aqueduct;

> **tectospinal tract**, which has arisen from superior colliculus and whose fibers have crossed in the **dorsal tegmental decussation**; tectospinal tract is just ventral to the medial longitudinal fasciculus and remains intimately proximate to it throughout brainstem;

superior cerebellar peduncles, which occupy much of the tegmentum at this level, on either side; they have not decussated at this level (we're lower, compared to last chapter);

central tegmental tract, whose white matter seems to blend into superior cerebellar peduncle on the latter's medial side;

spinothalamic and medial lemniscal tracts, ventral to **superior cerebellar peduncle**;
and, dorsolaterally, **lateral lemniscus**.

VENTRAL/BASAL NUCLEI. I'll quote Nauta and Feirtag (1986) once more, this time on the subject of the bluish nucleus mentioned a moment ago; the italics, again, are mine:

> The transmitter norepinephrine is employed by the *locus ceruleus*, a group of roughly 20,000 neurons extending from *the ventrolateral corner of the central gray substance some distance into the adjacent tegmentum . . ..* The region indeed is cerulean, or distinctly dark blue in color, both in fresh brains and in brains fixed in formaldehyde. The blueness reflects the region's content of neuromelanin, a pigment synthesized by most of the neurons of the *locus.* The pigment is a polymer of dihydroxyphenylalanine, or DOPA, the precursor of the catecholamine neurotransmitters. Apart from its chemical properties, the *locus ceruleus* is remarkable anatomically: its *efferents are distributed to all the main divisions of the central nervous system.* On average, then, its 20,000 neurons must each influence a very great number of neurons elsewhere in the brain. In that respect, *the locus ceruleus is a caricature of the reticular formation: it embodies the extreme expression of a prominent reticular trait, an apparent diffuseness and nonspecificity of synaptic connections.*

As in their discussion of central or periaqueductal grey, they allude to an aspect of brainstem anatomy that doesn't lend itself to a point-at-a-thing-and-name-it approach. *Diffuseness and nonspecificity of synaptic connections*: it's a concept worth elaborating now.

Certainly you can point to *locus ceruleus* in a gross specimen. As plain to the eye as that nucleus is, a largely unseen network–which calls to mind Camille Golgi's notion of branching arborization as a key to microanatomy (his reticularism, as opposed to Ramón y Cajal's neuronism [Jones, 1999 and Sterling, 1998])–is present throughout brainstem. We're not just talking about the reticular formation, whether mesencephalic or rhombencephalic. We also refer to a number of diffuse systems and their arbors.

Let's discuss three of them, all represented in the rostral pons.

We teach that *locus ceruleus* neurons synthesize norepinephrine. We say that **nuclei of the raphe**–the raphe being the seam or suture mentioned earlier–synthesize serotonin, an indolamine. We refer to a cholinergic zone (it seems to me more a zone than a nucleus; there are cholinergic neurons even in the central grey) in the lateral tegmentum of the high pons. A cholinergic **pedunculopontine nucleus** has been of interest in the modern treatment of Parkinson's disease, because long-term stimulation of the area may improve gait (Aravamuthan et al., 2007). All the anatomic-structural associations mentioned–*locus ceruleus* with norepinephrine, raphe nuclei with serotonin, and pedunculopontine nucleus with acetylcholine–are essentially correct, but they are simplifications compared to the true anatomy.

The *locus ceruleus* accounts for perhaps only 50% of neurons that synthesize norepinephrine; the remainder of catecholaminergic neurons are found in less discretely bounded locales through the pontine and medullary tegmentum. Although serotonergic neurons can be found in multiple nuclei that hug the midline raphe, not all raphe nuclear neurons are serotonergic; indeed, probably only a minority of neurons in many raphe nuclei are indolaminergic. Finally, cholinergic neurons don't occupy a neat grey unit either; they seem instead to be scattered not only in the area of pedunculopontine nucleus, but also in the so-called **medial and lateral parabrachial nuclei of rostral pons**.

We teach about projections from the above nuclei or zones to diverse locales–*efferents distributed to all the main divisions of the central nervous system*, per Nauta and Feirtag. Consider cholinergic axons:

> Cholinergic neurons . . . in the mesopontine reticular formation (particularly the pedunculopontine nucleus) compose the major excitatory reticulothalamic pathway to the nonspecific thalamocortical system; they influence this system by direct excitation of thalamocortical neurons, as well as by disinhibition of the thalamic reticular nucleus (Kinney and Samuels, 1994).

Studious attempts have been made to follow cholinergic projections to thalamus and elsewhere, but one wonders whether one loses a sense of the tree by obsessive attention to its branches.

That said, here are some basics regarding neurotransmitter projections from dispersed, high pontine locales:

Many, not all, cholinergic projections ascend in the **dorsal tegmental pathway,** also known as the **dorsal longitudinal fasciculus** (Shute and Lewis, 1967).

Many, not all, noradrenergic fibers ascend via the **central tegmental tract** and **median forebrain bundle** to cortical destinations (Nieuwenhuys, 1985).

Some, not all, serotonergic pass via **dorsal tegmental pathway** and **median forebrain bundle** to rostral points (Nieuwenhuys, 1985).

The pathways mentioned are typically bidirectional. So, hypothalamic axons also descend in the **dorsal tegmental pathway,** although there's debate over whether, for example, projections from parvocellular paraventricular nucleus of hypothalamus connect monosynaptically with neurons in the spinal cord's intermediolateral grey column, from whence second-order arise in the sympathetic pupillodilatory pathway (Carpenter and Sutin, 1983 and Burnstock, 2009).

VENTRAL/MOTOR NUCLEI. There are theories, but no one really knows what cortical information transmits via the **frontopontine** and **temporopontine tracts**–the bundles of Arnold and Türck, respectively–to **pontine nuclei.** Nor is it trivial to map those nuclei. There are clever people who have imported neuroimages of pontine infarctions into a Photoshop program to create topographies (maps) of rostral/basal motor fibers and nuclei, based on associated clinical deficits:

The syndromes are not absolutely discrete . . .. Structure-function correlations indicate that strength is conveyed by the corticofugal fibers destined for spinal cord, whereas dysmetria results from lesions involving the neurons of the basilar pons [*basis pontis*] that link the ipsilateral cerebral cortex with the contralateral cerebellar hemisphere (Schmahmann et al., 2004).

To quibble momentarily, the word corticofugal (*fugere*, Latin, to flee) needs some qualification. It's not that homolateral cortico-pontine fibers heading to contralateral cerebellar hemisphere, via pontine connections, aren't also fleeing cortex. They do. The authors want to distinguish between how damage to a certain population of fibers can result *in weakness* as opposed to how pontine-nuclear damage or a lesion of pontocerebellar fibers can result in *incoordination* that's disproportionate to whatever weakness there may be, if any. The distinction can be hard to judge, given the physical proximity of *both* corticofugal systems in the pons.

There are generalizations we can consider, based on the authors' correlations. In the rostral pons, facial strength is represented dorsomedially; articulation (the *coordination* of movements to produce speech) is ventromedial. Swallowing maps all through rostral pons, medially, laterally, and ventrally. In a very overlapping way, hand and arm strength and coordination map to ventral *basis pontis*. Note that we describe just the rostral pons for the time being.

*

Pontine nuclei: what *are* they? Based on studies in cats, two provocative theorists (Blomfield and Marr, 1970) talk about the one thing that they can confidently say about cortico-cerebellar intercommunication. By way of serial monosynaptic connections, it's fast:

. . . discharges in the pontine nuclei follow stimulation of the cerebral white matter by as little as 2 ms [milliseconds]. . . . Contextual information reaching the cerebellar cortex through the mossy fibres is also rapidly transmitted . . . .. The time taken for stimulation of the subcortical white matter to evoke a mossy fibre response is 2.7 ms.

If you're curious about other conduction in an informational loop that returns from cerebellum to cortex, the intervals are also speedy:

> . . . pontine nuclei to cerebellar nuclei, 1 ms [this projection exists, perhaps, to our surprise]; cerebellar nuclei to VL [ventrolateral] nucleus of thalamus, 2 ms; VL nucleus of thalamus to [deep, presumably layer V or Betz] cerebral pyramidal cells, an estimated 1 ms.

The role of pontine nuclei in the second passage seems more than the transfer of action potentials across the midline to contralateral cerebellum; projections from those nuclei to deep cerebellar nuclei hint at a positive feedback loop in which ". . . a movement–once initiated–will tend to continue indefinitely (at least well beyond the normal firing period of pyramidal cells in response to excitatory input): and this will only be terminated either by applying direct inhibition to the deep pyramidal cells or by breaking the feedback loop."

That the theory is old shouldn't worry us. It's of use to illustrate that pontine nuclei may be involved in moment-to-moment motor control. They aren't merely internuncial or connector neurons.

34

Properly in the Fourth Ventricle

Where the cerebral aqueduct once was in previous axial sections, now we visualize a widening quadrilateral space, which is the fourth ventricle. I imagine myself inside that ventricle, and I want to know what's above, below, and to the sides of me.

Don't forget **RULE #4**. We apply the following to all our axial sections: ventral brainstem is *below* dorsal brainstem. (In MR and CT images, unlike anatomic sections, ventral brainstem is above dorsal brainstem.)

I stand astride the midline suture or median sulcus that divides symmetrical halves of the pons; my feet are on the floor of the fourth ventricle. On either side of the midline (my feet barely apart), my feet touch the so-called median eminences, in modern anatomical parlance. But anatomists of a former time referred to round bundles, which are the **medial longitudinal fasciculi** inside the eminences. If I reach up to touch the fastigium (top) above me, my fingers touch the underside of the **superior medullary velum**, but dorsal to that velum is the most rostral– and rather tiny–lobule of the cerebellar *vermis*, the ***lingula***.

I seem to be under a kind of gambrel roof, because, to either side of my outstretched arms, the margins are at acute angles to the fourth ventricular floor. The superior cerebellar peduncles tent me dorsolaterally. These superior peduncles go by another name, the *brachia conjunctivae* (singular: ***brachium conjunctivum***).

A *brachium* is an arm. The Latin root of *conjuctivum* is a verb having to do with joining or connection. For example, the *conjunctiva of the eye* conjoins the eyeball surface to that of the inner eyelid. So, what does a *brachium conjunctivum* connect? In the 19th century, there was a thought about a bending commissure between deep cerebellar nuclei on one side and the inferior olive on the other (Voogd and van Baarsen, 2014). That's not the modern view, but it's interesting. Keep in mind that the central tegmental tract is very close to the tegmental *brachium conjunctivum* before the latter decussates. The **central tegmental tract** is a boulevard traversed by fibers from red nucleus to homolateral inferior olive. Add the contralateral **dentate nucleus** of cerebellum and you've identified the vertices of a **rubro-olivary-dentate triangle (of Guillain and Mollaret)**, lesions of which are associated with certain tremors or myoclonus.[4]

The oddity and interest of the superior cerebellar peduncle is its *dorsolateral* presence at the roof of the fourth ventricle, its *ventromedial* location in rostral pontine tegmentum, and thence to what we've called (in an appropriately stained section) a big blob of black in the midbrain tegmentum, i.e., the **decussation of superior cerebellar peduncles**. The superior cerebellar peduncle is the largest efferent tract leaving cerebellum; it's an arm that bends in space to reach across the midline. Its axons (say, in the right *brachium conjunctivum*) arise from (right) dentate nucleus, the most lateral of the (right) deep cerebellar nuclei. The (right) superior cerebellar peduncle connects (right) deep cerebellar nuclei with red nucleus and, mainly, with thalamus on the contralateral (left) side.

---

4   If (left) red nucleus, (left) inferior olive, and (right) dentate nucleus are the vertices, what are the sides of the triangle? (Left) red nucleus and (left) inferior olive connect via the central tegmental tract without fibers crossing the midline. (Right) dentate projects to (left) red nucleus via the superior cerebellar peduncle. There is a medullary olivocerebellar projection: (left) olivary fibers cross the midline in medulla to project to contralateral (right) dentate via the (right) inferior cerebellar peduncle (Ruigrok TJH and Voogd J, 2000), although there's controversy about whether the last of the three sides is relevant to the pathology of palatal myoclonus (Lapresle and Hamida, 1970).

It's been further observed that palatal myoclonus associated with lesions of the triangle is side-specific: myoclonus occurs on the side opposite lesions of the olive and central tegmental tract, but on the same side in cerebellar lesions (Gautier and Blackwood, 1961). From that 1961 paper (cases 2 and 3), twitching of the palate towards the right was associated with left inferior olivary changes in both, but right dentate pathology in case 2 and left central tegmental tract pathology in case 3.

Looking up at the dorsolateral roof of the fourth ventricle, I have no presentiment that the *brachium conjunctivum* will cross the midline: all I know is that the left *brachium* has arisen from left cerebellum, right *brachium* from right cerebellum. I'd have to track an axon in one peduncle along its entire course to convince myself that there's a crossing. In the eyes of Galen of Greek antiquity, the *brachium conjunctivum* simply looked like a "tendon" of brain; he didn't observe its decussating path (Voogd and van Baarsen, 2014). At the present level, one appreciates the early Greek observation.

*

I'm still standing inside the fourth ventricle. Gazing again at its floor, assuming that my view isn't obscured by choroid plexus or a lattice of vessels, I'm interested in the lateral edge, at the acutest angle formed by the floor and the slant gable of superior cerebellar peduncle above it. Neurosurgical colleagues would say that there's no obvious landmark there, certainly not as plain as the so-called facial colliculi on the fourth ventricular floor at a level caudal to where we are now. Anatomy colleagues might say that the **sulcus limitans** (described by Wilhelm His, Sr. in the 19th century; his son, the junior, described the bundle of His in the heart) isn't as clearly present anatomically here as it is, for example, in medulla.

Is it possible to distinguish alar from basal nuclei at our current level? Keep in mind that, in development, neurons might originate in basal plate, but they translocate to lateral positions by maturity (Puelles et al., 2018). Yet, at the very lateral corner of the fourth ventricle, here at the level of the **principal sensory and motor nuclei of CN V** (which are deep and lateral to the corner), the principal sensory nucleus *is dorsolateral* to the principle motor nucleus. There's also a bit of the **mesencephalic trigeminal nucleus** at the current level: applying the simplification that sensory nuclei are lateral to motor ones, we'd surmise that mesencephalic trigeminal nucleus is lateral to the principal motor nucleus–which it is.

In short, division into alar/dorsal/lateral (= sensory) and basal/ventral/ medial (= motor) might not be perfect, but it's a serviceable way of thinking about important brainstem nuclei. Note that the distinction we mentioned in midbrain–a division between alar/dorsal/sensory nuclei and basal/ ventral/motor nuclei–tilts its axis such that sensory nuclei are now *lateral* to motor nuclei.

Nieuwenhuys (2011) has strong views on the subject:

> According to His (1891, 1893) the brainstem consists of two longitudinal zones, the dorsal alar plate (sensory in nature) and the ventral basal plate (motor in nature). [John Black] Johnston and [C. Judson] Herrick [both Americans, who published in the very early 20th century] indicated that both plates can be subdivided into separate somatic and visceral zones, distinguishing somatosensory and viscerosensory zones with the alar plate, and visceromotor and somatomotor zones within the basal plate. . . . Recent developmental molecular studies on brains of birds and mammals confirmed the presence of longitudinal zones, and also showed molecularly defined transverse bands or neuromeres throughout development . . .. [I]t may be hypothesized that the brainstems of all vertebrates share a basic organizational plan, in which intersecting longitudinal and transverse zones form fundamental histogenetic and genoarchitectonic units.

All I want to do is keep organizing my anatomical information. At our current pontine level, the mesencephalic and principal sensory nuclei of CN V are lateral to the principal motor nucleus in the tegmentum.

Elsewhere in that tegmentum, ventral to the floor of fourth ventricle, we re-acknowledge the white matter tracts we've previously encountered:

> **medial longitudinal fasciculus** at the midline, below my feet;

> **tectospinal tract**, just below the medial longitudinal fasciculus, retaining its intimate proximity to it;

> **central tegmental tract**, which is less obvious than in higher sections;

> **spinothalamic and medial lemniscal tracts**, ventral to the central tegmental tract;
> and, dorsolaterally, **lateral lemniscus**;

the **pyramidal tracts** appear to be condensing into a discrete white-matter bundles in the ventral *basis pontis*.

VENTRAL/MOTOR PONTINE NUCLEI. Recall our Photoshop colleagues from the last chapter; we cite them again (Schmahmann et al., 2004). In the pons at the level of CN V nuclei, facial strength isn't much represented much at all; neither is articulation. Instead, strength maps to ventral *basis pontis* (where the pyramidal tract is, now more obviously than in more superior sections). Coordination of a leg maps to presumptive pontine nuclei located in dorsal and dorsolateral *basis pontis*; coordination of gait maps, frankly, all over the place: to the most ventral *basis pontis* at our previous (higher) level, our current one, and also caudal to our present level.

*

Regarding the conspicuous appearance of the **middle cerebellar peduncle**, to either side of the pons laterally, let's distill information about it:

a.   It's also called the ***brachium pontis***.

In axial section, one doesn't quite appreciate the sweeping course of the *brachia*.

Warning, here comes a gratuitous association. I think about a statue in the Louvre in Paris, from the Hellenistic period, named the Winged Victory of Samothrace. It's striking. Nine feet tall. It's a headless and armless woman, draped in flowing garments that draft against her body and behind her, as if in an oncoming wind. She has immense wings which extend behind her. If you stand directly in front of her (you gaze up, because she stands on a pedestal), the leading edge of the wings seem level with the shoulders; the wing feathers dangle down. In that one view of her outspread wings, I visualize the sweeping course of the medial cerebellar peduncles on either side of the pons.

b.   The middle cerebellar peduncle is the largest afferent pathway into cerebellum, "quantitatively the most important route by which the cerebral cortex can influence cerebellar cortex" (Carpenter and Sutin, 1983). Projections from much of cortex (frontal motor, dorsolateral prefrontal, parietal, and superior temporal–at least those locales) descend to pontine nuclei on the same side, then second-order axons in the middle cerebellar peduncle decussate into the medullary core of the contralateral cerebellar hemisphere.

c. In the pontine tegmentum, transversely oriented fibers that will make up the middle cerebellar peduncles pass both dorsal and ventral to the descending fibers of the pyramidal tract. The anatomic proximity of structures related to coordination and to strength makes one think that, here, ataxia and hemiparesis could simultaneously result from a discrete lesion. Nevertheless, regarding the case we discussed at the start of this seminar, a curious point arises: ". . . it is not clear why the cerebellar signs are not bilateral" (Fisher, 1978). What passes from left to right also passes from right to left, hence the question of why a unilateral lesion wouldn't result in bilateral signs.

35

Beyond Brazis

If you've forgotten who Brazis is (admittedly, our chapter 28 was a long time ago), he's the author of chapter 14 of *Localization in Clinical Neurology*. I return to his chapter now that we're half-way into our tour of axial brainstem sections. It's a reasonable moment to take stock of where we've been.

Here is Brazis's summary of an ataxic hemiparesis:

> ATAXIC HEMIPARESIS. A lesion (usually a lacunar infarction) in the basis pontis at the junction of the upper one-third and lower two-thirds of the pons may result in the ataxic-hemiparesis (homolateral ataxia and crural [related to the leg] paresis syndrome. In this syndrome hemiparesis, which is more severe in the lower extremity, is associated with ipsilateral hemiataxia and occasionally dysarthria, nystagmus, and paresthesias. The lesion is in the contralateral pons. This syndrome has also been has also been described with contralateral thalamocapsular lesions (Brazis, 1985).

Eighty-three words in length, the description is not only mercifully short, but also it repeats itself, I assume, for emphasis: ataxic hemiparesis is mentioned twice; then we have homolateral ataxia and *crural* paresis followed by an iterative description (hemiparesis, *which is more severe in the*

173

lower extremity, . . . associated with ipsilateral hemiataxia . . .). Then we get two possible localizations, both textbook. The one in brainstem is rather precise, at the junction of the upper one-third and lower two-thirds of the pons–which is about the location where we ended the preceding chapter. I take the paragraph to be of the tell-them-what-you-are-going-to-say-then-say-it-then-tell-them-what-you-just-said school of instruction.

Yet if I confidently talk about a left pontine localization for a right-sided ataxic hemiparesis, because Brazis echoes in my head, then I tacitly violate **RULES #1** and **#2**.

The 44 year-old man in our chapter 28 had no dysarthria, but a left-beating nystagmus, diminished optokinetic nystagmus (OKN) with leftward moving targets, and a sense that the right hand (only) was swollen or stiff, in the absence of a sensory deficit. Most of all, he had a motor problem that invites one "to postulate a single site along the cerebral neuraxis where pyramidal and cerebellar signs would not be contralateral to each other" (Fisher, 1978).

The authors whom I've affectionately called Photoshop colleagues (the lead author works across town) teach me the following, based on studies in monkeys:

> . . . pontocerebellar fibres from one side of the pons traverse the opposite hemipons, and disperse amongst numerous, widely divergent pontocerebellar fascicles before coalescing into the opposite brachium pontis. Together with the motor corticopontine projections that terminate in multiple discrete regions in the middle and caudal pons, this arrangement may account for the absence of ipsilateral dysmetria in all but the largest infarcts. In smaller lesions, sufficient numbers of pontocerebellar fibres from the intact hemipons escape damage as they bypass the lesion on their way to the cerebellum, thus preventing ipsilateral dysmetria (Schmahmann et al., 2004).

OK, but does nystagmus and a paresthetic sense of swollen-ness (in just the right hand) make one think of a larger area of ischemia? Likewise, why did the man have such a problem *with his right arm*–recall that he couldn't light his cigarette; and, on finger-to-nose testing, wild oscillations caused him to strike his own face. Did an ischemic penumbra extend into higher pons?

Is there anatomy that we haven't studied in enough depth to account for all the clinical findings, in the same way that we need to know about the ramification of pontocerebellar fibers before they coalesce in (contralateral) middle cerebellar peduncle to explain why the 44 year-old man's cerebellar findings aren't bilateral?

The OKN finding had me thinking at first about a parietal (supratentorial) lesion; loss of OKN can happen in brainstem disease, but one might expect an accompanying gaze palsy (Davidoff et al., 1966). The unidirectional, leftward beating nystagmus had me thinking at first about a right vestibular problem, but unidirectional nystagmus could also be a dysfunction of gaze-holding mechanisms in brainstem. The paresthetic right hand, if his sense of swelling or stiffness was a paresthesia, was significant to me simply because it was on the right side (I didn't know what to make of the sense, and he had no sensory deficit per se). All the above were lesser aspects of the presentation.

Regarding the ataxic hemiparesis itself (all its aspects, including falling to the right on Romberg testing), we repeat to ourselves that cerebellar and pyramidal tracts are closest to each other physically/anatomically in the midbrain or pons. Then we read how the original authors excluded the midbrain:

> If the responsible lesion were in the upper midbrain or subthalamic region it would be possible to involve the superior cerebellar peduncle after it has crossed the midline, and the cerebral peduncle lying immediately anterior to it, producing a combined cerebello-pyramidal disturbance on the opposite side. In our [case] . . . there were no signs of midbrain involvement such a third nerve palsy . . . (Fisher and Cole, 1965).

Why the right arm was so dyscoordinated still strikes me as curious. Perhaps the ischemia involved more rostral pons (where, perhaps, arm and hand are more generously represented, both in terms of strength and coordination), but, if so, one might have expected right arm weakness as well as bilateral cerebellar findings, given the larger affected territory.

We have no imaging or pathological correlation in the case.

*

To localize a lesion in left pons, at the junction of its upper one-third and lower two-thirds, is to invite consideration about how damage to certain structures rather than others disrupts what the brain is trying to accomplish in the first place.

Theorists talk about levels of analysis in trying to explain how the brain controls movement–the highest level relates to "the nature of the problem to be solved" (Alexander et al., 1994). In our patient's case, maybe the high-level problems included walking and lighting a cigarette. But certainly right now, I'm at a very low level of analysis, and, yes, there's always anatomy that we can study in greater depth. Nor can we comment about whatever computations in different systems result in a normal gait or a lit cigarette. All that we seek is: to remain aware of distinct structures that are close to each other. Maybe we can start to understand principles of organization based on the anatomy's divisible proximities, such as that between principal sensory and motor nuclei of CN V or the non-overlapping nearness of cerebellar and pyramidal tracts in midbrain or pons.

36

On the Facial Colliculus

June 17, 1858, a Thursday. A 43 year-old man, previously in good health except for a congenital atrophy of his right arm, had a restless night on the 16th. He didn't understand why he couldn't sleep. A bureaucrat of some type and apparently single, he earned enough money to satisfy his daily needs; he had a penchant for alcoholic beverages. He hadn't been ill recently. He recalled having a "brain fever" at age ten. In the early morning of the 17th, without cognizance of what had happened or how he got there, he was found down in the middle of a street. At first, he couldn't speak. He vomited copiously. By the time he got to hospital at 7 a.m., his mental state had cleared almost completely.

The first full examination we have dates to six days after his presentation. There were three findings: a right hemiparesis, a conjugate gaze paralysis looking to the left (both eyes couldn't look to the left in the horizontal plane), and a left facial paralysis–the last manifesting a smooth, unwrinkled left forehead, an inability to close the left eyelids, and an effaced left nasolabial fold.

I'll cite the source later. For now, I want to keep the case in mind as we continue our tour of axial sections.

*

We're still in pons. I'm standing again in the fourth ventricle, and I want to know, yet again, what's above, below, and to the sides of me.

I stand astride the midline suture or median sulcus that divides symmetrical halves of the pons; my feet are on the floor of the fourth ventricle. But my footing is curious here. I feel that I stand on large domes on either side of the midline, and that the whole floor of the fourth is now more undulated than previously. My left foot balances on the left facial colliculus; my right on the right colliculus. So, what are these colliculi; why are they reliably identifiable landmarks in endoscopy of the fourth ventricle (Longetti et al., 2008); why do they exist in the first place? Another way of asking the last question is: why do facial-nerve fascicles on either side loop around CN VI (abducens) nuclei? Fascicular CN VII doesn't loop at all in the oldest branch of vertebrates represented by the lamprey (Pombal and Megías, 2018), and the internal facial genu in frogs and birds is nothing like what it is in humans (Fritzsch, 1998). Here's a textbook answer:

> . . . the cell masses of the branchiomotor zone have migrated away from their original periventricular position. Their efferent fibers, however, have retained their original position. As a consequence, these fibers make a loop, directed at the floor of the fourth ventricle before they leave the brainstem in a lateral direction. In the case of the seventh nerve, this loop in known as the *genu* (knee) of the facial nerve. It can be recognized as an elevation in the floor of the fourth ventricle: the facial collicule [colliculus] (Nieuwenhuys et al., 2008).

Primordial facial branchiomotor neurons *move* from one place to another in development. They venture caudally to their mature location, inferior to CN VI nucleus (McKay et al., 1997), but I wonder whether migration, whose path *is* the facial nerve's internal genu if you envision moving lateral to medial (though the efferent fibers pass medial to lateral), understates what we see in front of us.

We discuss a particularly complicated cranial nerve and its likewise complex functional circuitry (Chandrasekhar et al., 1997), since CN VII isn't only branchiomotor. It doesn't only innervate branchial arch-derived muscles that control facial expression. It's also secretomotor in its innervation of lacrimal and salivary glands, as well as sensory, in how it transmits afferent taste from the anterior two-thirds of the tongue as well as skin sensation from the ear's pinna and external auditory meatus.

Facial motor nucleus (branchiomotor), **superior salivatory nucleus** (secretomotor), **nucleus of the solitary tract** (taste), and **spinal trigeminal nucleus** (sensation of outer ear) are responsible for their respective CN VII functions (Chandrasekhar, 2004). And if you follow the course of fascicular CN VII from its motor nucleus (caudal to CN VI nucleus) to the genu at the facial colliculus (where axons wrap around abducens nucleus at the facial collicule) to its exit at the pontomedullary junction, you find yourself at various points close to the discrete brainstem nuclei involved in all CN VII modalities.

*

Note to self: if there's a superior salivatory nucleus, there must be an inferior one, right? Not necessarily, as I read in Carpenter and Sutin (1983):

> [Superior salivatory nucleus is a] poorly defined nucleus . . .. Retrograde transport studies indicate that preganglionic parasympathetic neurons form an uninterrupted dorsal cell column extending from the medulla into the pons. Cells of the dorsal motor nucleus of the vagus form the more caudal portion of this column; cells in the more rostral regions are less compact and distributed over a wide region of the reticular formation. In the pons cells of this column lie between the nucleus of the solitary tract and the facial motor nucleus. The overlapping origins of neurons contributing to the glossopharyngeal [CN IX] and intermediate nerve [that portion of CN VII carrying afferent sensory and efferent secretomotor fibers] raises a question concerning the appropriateness of a nomenclature that distinguishes separate salivatory nuclei as inferior and superior.

Is the above too much information? No, and here's why: note the phrase *uninterrupted dorsal cell column*. We turn to columns soon.

*

There's more to say about structures bounded within the dome of facial colliculus. The round bundle or medial longitudinal fasciculus still hugs the midline, as it did in our last, more rostral axial section. Then, there's the simply non-trivial matter of **CN VI (abducens) nucleus** and its connections.

I plainly see the nucleus; the internal facial genu wraps around it. But I know that it's intimately associated with **paramedian pontine reticular formation**, about which several observations come to mind:

1. It's not readily visualized (it's reticular);
2. It's present both at the level of CN VI nucleus and above/rostral to CN VI nucleus;
3. If you can't readily visualize it, how do you know where it is? In young monkeys, stimulation by an electrode passed from rostral to caudal in brainstem resulted in (Cohen et al., 1968):
   a. vocalization (at the level of central grey matter surrounding aqueduct of Sylvius);
   b. depression of one eye in adduction (intorsion of the eye contralateral to the site of stimulation) at the level of CN IV nucleus;
   c. adduction of one eye (the eye ipsilateral to the site of stimulation) at the level of medial longitudinal fasciculus above CN VI nucleus);
   d. conjugate, ipsilateral, horizontal eye movements when in the paramedian pontine reticular formation (if stimulation on the left, then both eyes look horizontally to the left);
5. It's involved in gaze holding;
6. If you *lesion* it (say, in the left paramedian pontine reticular formation), you cause paresis or paralysis of conjugate, ipsilateral, horizontal gaze (both eyes can't look horizontally to the left).

So, how do you differentiate between a lesion of (left) paramedian pontine reticular formation, a lesion of (left) CN VI nucleus itself, a lesion of fascicles emerging from (left) CN VI but still within the pons, and a (left) CN VI palsy?

The four parts of the question yield four distinct answers, each of which requires anatomical information.

Regarding (left) **paramedian pontine reticular formation**, I read that it's "the final prenuclear anatomical substrate for ipsilateral saccades" (Daroff et al., 1990). What do those words mean *in detail*? With respect to a cortically directed horizontal saccade of both eyes *to the left*, one typically invokes the so-called frontal eye field *in right cortex*–roughly, the posterior portion of the right middle frontal gyrus. One could also talk about a role for *right* superior colliculus as well, since right frontal eye field also projects to right superior colliculus by way of so-called direct and indirect basal ganglionic pathways.

Decussation of the corticobulbar pathway to left brainstem is said to happen somewhere in the reticular formation, either at the level of low midbrain or upper pons. At the level of the decussation, we are supra- or pre-nuclear, relative to CN VI nucleus. The corticobulbar projection, specifically with respect to our horizontal saccade of both eyes to the left, terminates in left paramedian pontine reticular formation, which is the location of excitatory burst neurons that project to two types of CN VI neurons. A lesion in paramedian pontine reticular formation–and one has as yet really to describe [left] CN VI nucleus–results in a paralysis of conjugate lateral gaze to the left.

(Left) **CN VI nucleus** isn't same as the paramedian pontine reticular formation. Fascicles leaving the nucleus emerge from its medial aspect en route to their exit as the abducens nerve at ventral pons. (In an appropriately stained axial section, it's easy to confuse CN VI fascicles as part of the internal facial genu, but those two differ, of course.) The nucleus contains not only motoneurons related to its control of the lateral rectus muscle, but also internuclear neurons whose fibers cross the midline roughly at the level of (left) CN VI nucleus to ascend in right medial longitudinal fasciculus. To repeat, interneurons inside (left) CN VI nucleus receive excitatory bursts from the (left) paramedian pontine reticular formation just as the motoneurons do.

The nucleus *receives* afferents not only from (left) pontine paramedian reticular formation, but also: from the (left) inner ear vestibule via (left) medial vestibular nucleus, (left) vestibular sensory ganglion of Scarpa (which is uniquely situated within CN VIII), and from the nucleus prepositus hypoglossi, which we'll discuss when we get to medulla.

Daroff et al. (1990) write that ". . . a unilateral lesion of the sixth nucleus produces an ipsilateral gaze palsy"; *both* eyes can't move to the left, because we know about interneurons inside CN VI nucleus. The authors make a further point, specifically with respect to a CN VI nuclear lesion, that "the *almost obligate* ipsilateral facial palsy, caused by involvement of the facial nerve fascicle dorsal to the nucleus, *provides the only reliable*

clinical means of distinguishing this gaze palsy from that produced by a PPRF
[paramedian pontine reticular formation] lesion at the same level [my italics]."

Next, regarding **fascicles emerging from (left) CN VI but still within
the pons**, Carpenter and Sutin (1983) write: "[t]he abducens [nucleus]
appears to be the only motor cranial nerve in which disturbances with
lesions of root fibers and nucleus are not identical." Here's why: a nuclear
lesion looks like a lesion of the paramedian pontine reticular formation,
not like a mononeuropathy affecting (left) lateral rectus in isolation. And,
as we just read, a nuclear lesion characteristically involves the fascicles of
the facial genu, hence the complete facial palsy described in the case that
began this chapter. From the original 1858 report, we read:

> . . . while he tries to move both or each separately, the eyes
> at once appear in the middle of the interpalpebral space to
> stop without being able to pass over [to the left] (Foville,
> 1858, translation by Silverman et al., 1995).[5]

And, yes, his left face was paralyzed as if he had a Bell's palsy.

The CN VI fascicle or central rootlet leaving the medial side of the
nucleus passes through the entire pontine tegmentum and *basis pontis*
before it exits the brainstem. A fascicular CN VI lesion, like a fascicular
CN VII lesion, shares many clinical aspects of an extra-axial cranial nerve
palsy. But given that the fascicle *en passant* keeps company with many other
structures, a (left) pontine lesion can produce signs in addition to a (left)
lateral rectus palsy, like a contralateral (right body) hemiparesis among
many other possible findings.

Regarding **an isolated (left) CN VI palsy**, we'd expect an isolated
paresis of (left eye) abduction in the horizontal plane without an associated
adduction problem in the right eye.

*

---

[5]   For the record, the Foville in question, author of the 1858 case, was Achille
Louis François Foville (1832-1887), not his father, who was Achille Louis
Foville (1799-1878). Both were anatomists and clinicians (Brogna et al.,
2012).

You're interested to address how the third of three findings from the 1858 case, the hemiparesis in the *right* body, links up with the first two findings, which we've discussed to the point of mild tedium.

Be patient.

*

We're still standing atop the facial colliculi. Indeed you're wondering if we ever plan to move elsewhere. Yet from this vantage point, thinking truly three dimensionally (**RULE #3**), we can appreciate the great deal that's all around us.

I'm interested in what might be lateral to the facial colliculus, moving across the floor of the fourth ventricle. The dome of the facial colliculus ends. At its lateral base angle, there's another mound extending to the gambrel roof that rises towards the fastigium (top) of the fourth ventricle above me. That lateral mound, described as a vestibular triangle (Nauta and Feirtag, 1986), contains, yes, vestibular nuclei.

There's a tendency for some to think of vestibular nuclei as being located just in the medulla. They're there in fact, but a column created by vestibular nuclei (no less than four nuclei) extends rostrally to our current level of pons. Since a fundamental task of the vestibular system is to control eye movements relative to the head's position in space, it makes sense that vestibular nuclei would be anatomically close to sites we've already discussed relevant to saccades and gaze.

I like to think much more simply: the vestibular nuclear column that extends, without interruption, from medulla to pons is . . . sensory. Anatomists say that the vestibular axons from vestibular nuclei are the most widely dispersed special sensory system in the neuraxis–the axons dispatch themselves to brainstem motor nuclei (especially those having to do with eyes), to cerebellum (especially vestibulocerebellum[6] or the *flocculus* and *nodulus*), to spinal cord, and to thalamus thence to cortex (Carpenter and Sutin, 1983 and Nieuwenhuys et al., 2008), but the nuclei themselves live in a single, discrete column.

Deep and lateral to the vestibular-nuclear column in the vestibular triangle, might we expect to find another sensory nucleus? Yes: **the spinal**

---

[6]   Rather than vestibulocerebellum, some anatomists prefer the term oculomotor cerebellum, which consists of more than just *flocculus* and *nodulus*.

tract and nucleus of CN V–it's a structure that we can track caudally into medulla and to cervical spinal cord (basically, it's a column).

Medial to spinal tract and nucleus of CN V, and medial to the vestibular nuclear column, would we expect other sensory nuclei? No, not if you're a proponent of a limiting sulcus that divides motor from sensory nuclei in pons. Instead, you'd expect motor nuclei, among them CN VI and CN VII motor nuclei (CN V motor nucleus is also medial, but it's located in the higher pons, as discussed in the last chapter) and **superior salivatory nucleus**, which is secreto*motor*. You find them where they, um, belong.

*

If I reach up to touch the fastigium (top) above me, previously my fingers touched the underside of the superior medullary velum and the *lingula* above it, but, now, buried in an expanse of white matter are **deep cerebellar nuclei**, the largest and most lateral of which is the **dentate nucleus**. Depending on the transverse section, perhaps a bit of vestibulocerebellar *nodulus* pokes into the dorsal space of fourth ventricle above my head.

To either side of my outstretched arms, the margins of the ventricle still angle inwards, relative to the undulated fourth ventricular floor. Yet, it's not just the superior cerebellar peduncle/*brachium conjunctivum* and middle cerebellar peduncle/*brachium pontis* that envelop me here. Once I visualize in my head the vestibular nuclear cell column in the vestibular triangle, since I know that some vestibular efferents from all four vestibular nuclei pass to cerebellum, I know I'm in the vicinity of the **juxtarestiform body**, through which those vestibulocerebellar fibers pass.

The juxtarestiform body lies at the dorsomedial edge of the **restiform body** or **inferior cerebellar peduncle**. (In a lateral view of an intact brainstem at the level of the medulla, the inferior cerebellar peduncle resembles a rope or, in Latin, a *restis* that passes from spinal cord upwards towards cerebellum, hence the alternative name.)

It's only in the pons where you visualize all three cerebellar peduncles in one transverse section. All three peduncles can be found in the white matter that I touch with my laterally outstretched arms.

*

Ventral to the floor of fourth ventricle, we re-acknowledge white matter tracts we've already encountered:

> **medial longitudinal fasciculus** at the midline, below my feet;
>
> **tectospinal tract**, just below the medial longitudinal fasciculus, retaining its intimate proximity to it;
>
> **central tegmental tract**;
>
> **spinothalamic and medial lemniscal tracts**, ventral to the central tegmental tract;
> and, dorsolaterally, **lateral lemniscus**;
> the **pyramidal tracts** in the ventral *basis pontis*.

There's something almost too obvious about the pons:

> The pons itself is riddled with fascicles. The transverse ones are pontocerebellar fibers, which cross the midline to join the contralateral brachium pontis. The longitudinal ones are corticopontine, corticobulbar, and corticospinal. The tegmentum–the dorsal division of the section–includes motor nuclei, sensory cell groups, and the reticular core of the section. It also includes nearly all of the brainstem's long fiber systems (Nauta and Feirtag, 1986).

I think that a conscientious student has some sense about which tracts run up and down as opposed to side to side, but there are opportunities to become confused. In an axial section in which white matter stains darkly, two transversely oriented black smears on either side of the midline separate the dorsal pontine tegmentum from the ventral *basis pontis*. In real anatomical dimensions, the thick white matter of those smears can be found just 0.75 centimeters below the floor of the fourth ventricle. Their transverse orientation shouldn't confuse, because we know that the **medial lemniscus** changes its axis during its winding brainstem course (in the pons it is transverse), but it's a longitudinal fiber system and an

185

obvious pontine structure. But the black smears aren't exclusively the medial lemnisci.

Less anatomically obvious is the **anterolateral fasciculus** (the **spinothalamic tract**), which is just lateral to the medial lemniscus; it, too, is a longitudinal fiber system. The **lateral lemniscus**, also a longitudinal fiber system and also found (dorso)lateral to medial lemniscus, heads to **inferior colliculus** in the auditory pathway. Yet the **trapezoid body** runs from side to side: its fibers cross the midline transversely and bidirectionally just at the place (or, ever so slightly inferior to) where we visualize the medial lemnisci as sideways smears. The trapezoid body is also part of the auditory pathway, and its anatomical presence introduces a curiosity in any attempt to organize one's thinking about the brainstem along the lines of a basal and alar plate division.

*

A few paragraphs ago, I asked, "Medial to spinal tract and nucleus of CN V, and medial to the vestibular nuclear column, would we expect other sensory nuclei?" I said that we wouldn't. But now consider a nucleus that is related and very proximate to the trapezoid body.

Buried in the stained, white-matter blackness of trapezoid body is a **superior olive**. I've traced the auditory pathway more completely in our second seminar, but for our present purposes, let me note: a. the superior olive is a key nucleus that receives auditory information from both cochleae; b. in an atlas of human brainstem, the superior olive can be hard to point to; c. I had never understood how it looked like an olive (such as the inferior olive) until I looked into the auditory pathways of mammals like bats, cats, or dogs. In the cat, for example, there's no mistaking a resemblance between superior olive and inferior olive. A convoluted, twisting shape of superior olivary nucleus is found in some mammals, but not in humans (Moore, 1987 and Nieuwenhuys et al., 2008).

The superior olive–actually, it's a complex of nuclei–is *medial* to the facial motor nucleus in the pontine tegmentum. Isn't it a sensory nucleus as CN VIII is a sensory nerve? Nieuwenhuys (2011) describes superior olive as a center of higher order. Is he blurring a basal-alar division that he takes so seriously?

*

Warning, I end this long chapter with an aside based on a dated reference (Irving and Harrison, 1967).

What possesses someone to perform a study in 49 mammals representing 14 species in which, among other goals, one wants to compare, for each species, the number of cells in a subnucleus of superior olive against the number of cells in CN VI nucleus? It turns out that there's a linear relationship, most convincing (my opinion) in animals with predominantly rod retinas, between the number of cells in medial superior olivary subnucleus and in CN VI nucleus. The authors factored nuclear diameters in relation to thickness of sections to arrive at estimated neuronal numbers. In the cat (large medial superior olive; rod retina), for example, there are about 1,000 neurons in CN VI nucleus and over 4,000 in medial superior olive. In the rat (small medial superior olive; rod retina), by comparison, there are roughly 200 neurons in CN VI nucleus compared to 700 in medial superior olive.

In animals with cone foveas or retinas, there's a similar linear relationship: the greater the number of superior olivary neurons, the greater the number of neurons in CN VI nucleus. In the macaque (large medial superior olive, cone fovea), the numbers are: roughly 4,500 CN VI neurons and just under 3,500 medial superior olivary neurons.

In ten species with rod retinas, there's no linear relationship between cell counts in CN VI nucleus and different auditory nucleus, located in trapezoid body.

The linear relationship specifically with respect to superior olive, the authors wrote, support a notion that there's an aspect of the auditory system ". . . probably concerned with the control of the visual apparatus by the location (and probably other aspects) of sounds. This system is present in animals with large eyes and may be regarded as a visual auditory system, having evolved as an adjunct of vision."

Is the quote a description of higher-order processing? One starts to wonder what a sensory nucleus really is—or in what way some nuclei would be best designated as sensorimotor.

37

What About the Weakness?
L'hémiplégie alterne[7]

At last, what's to be made of the 43-year-old man's right hemiparesis together with his conjugate left gaze palsy and left facial palsy? I want us to think . . . long before we blurt the words "left pons."

Recall from last chapter that the man's event happened early in the morning on June 17, 1858. By June 29, twelve or so days later, the gaze palsy and facial weakness were unchanged, but his right hemiparesis improved such that he could walk without help. The patient had an atrophy of the right arm antedating his event, so Foville was tentative to conclude much about the arm. I can't find a comment or hint about a sensory disturbance at any point.

My French is passable enough to read that crossed hemipareses (right body, left face or vice versa) had been discussed at the Paris Anatomical Society for some years before 1858. The pons had been contemplated as the site of causative lesions in *l'hemiplegie alterne* by many, including Poisson,

---

[7]   Weakness doesn't alternate from one side of the body to the other, as it does in, say, in the alternating hemiplegia of childhood, a pediatric genetic syndrome. It's a bit unfortunate that some authors talk about Foville and other eponymic brainstem syndromes as "alternating hemipareses" (e.g., Carpenter and Sutin, 1983). As Foville specifies, *alterne* really means "*une paralysie d'un côté du corps et du côté opposé de la face* [a paralysis of one side of the body and the opposite side of the face]."

Sénac, Millard, Gubler, Grenet, and perhaps even in his own father's textbook, from which Foville quotes.

Fast forward to this century and my hospital. Colleagues published a teaching case in 2006 (Selvadurai et al., 2006), in which we read that a 68-year-old man with a pontine telangiectasia on anticoagulation developed a left conjugate gaze palsy and right hemiparesis. In an accompanying video, the right arm is obviously weak and a left conjugate gaze palsy is also clear. There's no comment about the leg. There's no left facial paresis. Imaging showed an acute pontine hemorrhage extending dorsally and to the left. The left facial colliculus seems in the territory of the bleed. In a hemorrhage, you could argue that blood, unlike an ischemic infarction, might spare some structures, perhaps the left internal facial genu in particular.

Question: there's no pathological correlation to Foville's case, so how does one definitively explain *either* an incomplete presentation (as in 2006) *or* the complete one of 1858?

*

Let's speculate that the 43 year old suffered just a right monoparesis of the leg (which improved), just as the 68 year old seems to exhibit just a right arm monoparesis. Or, let's say that the 43 year old acutely suffered both arm and leg weakness, even if Foville couldn't tell with certainty because of the congenital deficit. Can we address the anatomy in all three permutations?

Given that somatotopic organization can be found in many nuclei and tracts throughout the neuraxis, the results of a prospective study correlating clinical and imaging findings might surprise:

> Despite the high number of pontine infarctions, we could not find any significant difference in pontine lesion location between patients with a predominantly arm paresis and those with a predominantly leg paresis. There was an area significantly affected by lesions causing arm predominant hemiparesis in the pons, but the lesions causing leg paresis appeared to be located above, within, and below it . . . (Marx et al., 2005).

The authors were interested in patients with acute oculomotor disorders, cranial nerve dysfunction, and limb or gait abnormalities suggestive of acute posterior circulation dysfunction. They recruited 258 consecutive patients; all were MR imaged within 48 hours of their events. Forty-one were diagnosed with something aside from a brainstem infarction.

Of the remaining 217, 155 had MR-diagnosed brainstem infarcts. Among the 155, 44 suffered an acute motor hemiparesis; 111 did not. Three of the 44 had multiple brainstem infarcts and were excluded. The remaining 41, all with isolated lesions and motor hemipareses, were used for correlation analysis. Clinically ascertained deficits were also studied with motor-evoked-potential studies within a week of presentation, save in three instances.

Of 41 motor hemipareses, arm weakness (more than leg) occurred in 20, leg weakness (more than arm) in 7; in 14 cases, arm and leg weakness were comparable. Three-dimensional image reconstructions and statistical analysis found: in a comparison of the 111 patients without hemiparesis and the 41 with hemiparesis, ventromedial, upper pontine lesions correlated with contralateral weakness of all types. Arm weakness mapped to pons at a level a bit superior to the level of the facial colliculus. Leg weakness mapped to levels above, at, and below the arm region.

We don't know much about the components of *l'hémiplégie alterne* in individual cases. All we know is that 14 of 41 had a facial paresis; 8 of 41 had some form of unspecified oculomotor disorder. We don't know how many had facial paresis and a conjugate gaze palsy together.

In their discussion, the authors sound ever so slightly apologetic: ". . . at least a moderate degree of corticospinal tract somatotopy is still maintained in the pons" even if (quoting from earlier in the text) "based on primate lesion studies . . . topographic arm/leg distribution appears to be progressively lost as the descending [corticospinal] tract traverses the pons."

They arrived at conclusions they didn't expect.

Save for arm paresis (maybe), pontine localization at a specific level based on weakness alone isn't as precise as the localization of a (left) conjugate lateral gaze palsy. And even a lesion at (left) facial colliculus can still produce an incomplete syndrome, as the 2006 teaching case attests.

*

The correlation paper is refreshing, because it reminds us that clinical data are . . . just what they are. When studying textbook anatomy, it's easy to be interrupted by Monday-morning questions, among them (my curt responses are in brackets):

Why wouldn't there be facial sensory manifestations and contralateral hemibody sensory manifestations in Foville's *l'hémiplégie alterne*? [Maybe there were.]

Could the hemiparesis in the 43 year old have been an ataxic hemiparesis (which improved)? [Yes.]

Why wasn't there even a suggestion of left facial paresis in the teaching case from 2006? [We've kinda answered that one.]

Assuming the 1858 case was an ischemic stroke, how large was the ischemic territory? [We'll never know.]

If it's true that somatotopy fractures (becomes somehow disorganized) in the pons, why is that? [Dunno. For that matter, why is there fractured somatotopy all through the cerebellum?]

Even if hemiparesis had not been present in the 43 year old's case, there's reason to believe that A.L.F. Foville, all of 26 years old and a year out of medical school, would still have written his paper. The first words of his publication's title reveal his almost naive, absolutely central interest: *Note sur une paralysie peu connue de certains muscles de l'œil* . . . [Note on a little-known paralysis of some muscles of the eye]. He had no knowledge of the paramedian pontine reticular formation and its burst neurons, of the two types of neurons in CN VI nucleus, and, most importantly, he had no familiarity with the medial longitudinal fasciculus, because its existence was unknown at the time. He was fascinated by the conjugate gaze palsy.

Pons associated with *l'hémiplégie alterne* was old hat to him.

*

We can amplify *alterne* to apply to brainstem as a whole, not just to pons.

A _____ of one side of the body and a _____ on the opposite side of the face makes one think about a brainstem localization, for which, as always, there are three possible answers.

"Face" means almost anything about it: the (left) eye, (left) pupil, (left) eyelid, the (left and right) eyes (looking to the left), (left) facial strength or sensation, (left) palate, (left) tongue, or what have you. And the contralateral hemibody findings are no less possibly diverse: (right) paresis, (right) ataxia, (right) paresthesiae, (right) sensory loss, (right) tremor, or what have you.

You want to see some *alterne* aspect to localize a lesion in brainstem, but findings especially in the face allow you, as a matter of principle, to increase your 0.333 likelihood of diagnostic success to a number approximating one.

38

Folded Grey Mass

The moment I visualize even a part of the folded grey mass that is **inferior olive**, I know that I'm in medulla. This chapter's title is from Brodal (1981). He reminds us that we refer to an obvious *collection of neurons* in the neighborhood of (depending on the cut, dorsal or lateral to) the medullary pyramid.

Not all axial sections in atlases are perfectly transverse. At the pontomedullary junction, which is our location now, sometimes you see just a sliver of inferior olive on one side but not the other. Not to worry.

RULE #7: If inferior olive anywhere, then medulla there.

I've seen students confuse inferior olive with another folded grey mass found in the vast, deep cerebellar white matter dorsal to the fourth ventricle. The latter grey matter is dentate nucleus, which we've encountered previously. There's reason to associate dentate nucleus and inferior olive in one's mind, because one could consider inferior olive as a ventrally displaced cerebellar nucleus (Kahle, 1986).

Pause. Think back to output from cerebellum:

The superior cerebellar peduncle is the largest efferent tract leaving cerebellum; it's an arm that bends in space to reach across the midline. Its axons (say, in the right *brachium conjunctivum*) arise from (right) dentate nucleus, the most lateral of the (right) deep cerebellar nuclei. The (right) superior cerebellar peduncle connects (right) deep cerebellar nuclei with red nucleus and, mainly, with thalamus on the contralateral (left) side.

The dentate is an important output nucleus (output from cerebellum via superior cerebellar peduncle a.k.a. *brachium conjunctivum*, to contralateral brain). The inferior olive is also an output nucleus–this chapter helps to fill the following blank–to contralateral _____?

*

The inferior olive is conspicuous. In humans, it's . . . beautiful.

Let's elaborate. The **principal nucleus of inferior olive** is especially well developed in humans, much more so than in a rat or cat (Baizer et al., 2011). There are two other subdivisions of inferior olive, including a dorsal accessory olive and a medial accessory olive, but I'll discuss the principal nucleus in particular. Its infoldings and sheer size distinguish it from other grey structures of brainstem. Thinking in three dimensions, an old anatomist described it as a crumpled purse whose opening is the **hilus**.

White matter cloaks the principal nucleus: the **central tegmental tract** "forms a fleece of myelinated fibres around the olive" (Nieuwenhuys et al., 2008); the fleece is the inferior olive's *amiculum* (cloak).

*

Perhaps you've noticed that textbook diagrams of cerebellar Purkinje cells depict just one climbing fiber per Purkinje cell. The origin of the one climbing fiber per Purkinje cell is inferior olive. Here's a good description:

> The fibers arising from the inferior olive end by branching on to the main neurons of the cerebellar cortex[,] called the Purkinje cells. These are the largest nerve cells in the brain, and the ends of the inferior olive axons, termed climbing fibers, literally climb up over the Purkinje cells' branching dendrites (fingerlike projections providing additional surface), where neurons receive input from other neurons (Llinás, 2001).

Other input to the Purkinje dendritic tree–by way of mossy fibers, not climbing fibers–includes, for example, cerebral cortical input via pontine nuclei and middle cerebellar peduncle. (Recall again from chapter 34: the middle cerebellar peduncle is the largest afferent pathway into cerebellum, "quantitatively the most important route by which the cerebral cortex can influence cerebellar cortex.") Purkinje axons, in turn, project to deep cerebellar nuclei, the dentate being the largest among them.

What's to be made of an architectural similarity between cerebral cortex, cerebellar cortex, the (highly folded) principal nucleus of inferior olive, and (also highly folded) dentate nucleus? Baizer et al. (2011) wonder about an evolutionary significance to involution or convolution of grey matter: ". . . human IOpr [principal nucleus of inferior olive] is reminiscent of the expansion of both cerebral and cerebellar cortex, both of which remain sheets with the development of sulci and gyri and a complex folding pattern. The increase in folding in the IOpr is similar to what is seen in the human dentate nucleus. Cerebral and cerebellar cortex, the IOpr, and the dentate nucleus all show complex folding patterns [in humans] . . .."

Not all grey matter structures involute, as Rakic (1995) pondered: cortical surface area increases by orders of magnitude from mouse to human, but cortical thickness only doubles between the species; then, if one compares the macaque monkey and human, asks Rakic, "What is the explanation for the approximately 15-fold larger number of postmitotic cells becoming distributed in the form of a thin, regular [folded] sheet rather than in a lump or globe, as has occurred during enlargement of the neostriatum over the same evolutionary period?"

The skeptic asks: so what?

The anatomist says: foldedness isn't just beautiful; it's very human.

In a pathway we'll trace in a moment, principal nucleus of inferior olive projects to cerebellar hemisphere, specifically to Purkinje cells. Brodal (1981) begs to differ about a one-to-one relationship between olivary and cerebellar cells: "It is often stated that there is a specific relation of one climbing fiber to one Purkinje cell. . . .. [A]natomically, branching of climbing fibers has been seen only in or just beneath the [cerebellar] cortex, and these branches supply two, three, or four Purkinje cells not far removed from each other. . . physiological investigations show that a single climbing fiber may branch and supply folia that are considerable distances apart." It appears that I've mis-taught all these years about one climbing fiber per Purkinje cell–maybe an excusable error.

What route do inferior olivary axons take to become climbing fibers specific to Purkinje cells?

*

The reader has noticed that I idiosyncratically situate myself in places like fourth ventricle. In the medulla, I'll start inside the **anterior median fissure**, my head above/dorsal to my feet. It's a tight space. I'm curious to know what's dorsal to my head and what's close to the midline on either side on me, and I'll try to visualize structures all the way up to the floor of the fourth ventricle.

We've not encountered the anterior median fissure. Neither have we really seen the medullary pyramids themselves, because the advent of a pyramid as a visible enlargement of ventroanterior funiculus *means* the medulla, along with the appearance of inferior olive lateral to pyramid. Because the ventroanterior funiculi on the ventral surface of medulla so robustly enlarge, the anterior median fissure between pyramids results, and that fissure extends all the way caudal/down to the point where it's briefly effaced by the decussation of the pyramids at the cervicomedullary junction.

Inside the anterior median fissure, to the immediate right and left of me, are the pyramids, but not just the pyramids.

Warning, here's a digression, but worth the trouble. In an appropriately stained section, the pyramids are black (all white matter), but there's space around the pyramids that isn't black. In fact, there are also *nuclei* to the immediate left and right of me in the anterior median fissure. In the spirit of "what *is* that?" I looked into those **arcuate nuclei**, which really do bend (*arcurare*) from the medial aspect of the pyramid, then ventral to it, then lateral to it.

Come to discover that the arcuate nuclei could be part of a medullary serotonergic network involved in control of the internal milieu, particularly its respiratory aspects (Kinney et al., 2011). For all the time in my life spent listening to patterns of breath in stuporous or comatose patients, I had no idea whatsoever about a role for nuclei I barely noticed in my books. You can see for yourself in a good atlas: they're obviously there.[8]

*

A midline seam dividing left and right halves of medulla points directly at the top of my head. On either side of the seam are white matter tracts that are, at a glance, parallel to the seam. Their fibers run from below to above where I stand at this axial level. The **medial lemniscus**, as we know, changes axis along its ribbon-like course heading rostrally. Here the medial lemnisci are upright, if you glean my meaning. I've characterized the medial lemnisci in my classes as a headless person standing on the pyramids–headless, because there's no representation of the head at our current level; arm representation in either lemniscus is above leg (arm higher than leg in each hemibody representation). Such are the up-standing medial lemnisci, but if I think carefully, the white matter above me can't just be passing in the caudal to rostral direction. There's a cross-weave of fibers above me.

Dorsolateral to the pyramid on either side is the principal nucleus of inferior olive, whose hilus points towards the midline. Inferior olivary axons emerge from the hilum, and pass transversely–for illustration, from

---

[8] To illustrate how widespread arcuate nuclear connections might be, try a dissection:

Look at the dorsal side of a medulla, particularly at the lower/caudal half of the fourth ventricle tented by the **inferior medullary velum**. Remove that velum to examine the floor of the fourth ventricle. You'll see a variable number of transversely running fibers which mark a kind of horizontal midline between the upper fourth ventricle and the end of the fourth ventricle, the latter called the *obex*.

The beautiful lateral strands, first observed by Piccolomini in the 16th century (Swanson, 2015), have been thought to be acoustic or cerebellar in nature, but a tracer study (Zec et al., 1997) suggests that arcuate nuclei project up the midline raphe and on to the floor of the fourth ventricle as these **medullary striae of Piccolomini**. The striae end in the vicinity of the inferior cerebellar peduncles at the level of the **foraminae of Luschka**. Also from the arcuate nuclei, passing superficially and laterally over the pyramids and olives, so-called **external arcuate fibers** end at much the same lateral place. Exposure to cerebrospinal fluid (for both projections) might relate to the homeostatic function of the network.

(right) hilus, *across* (right) medial lemniscus, then across the midline seam, then *across* (left) medial lemniscus. The fibers travel at right angles to the up-down fibers of the lemnisci, heading to contralateral destinations. Where?

Verbose answers:

1. The fibers traverse to (left) **inferior cerebellar peduncle**, a.k.a. the (left) **restiform body**, which is present very laterally at our axial level. The inferior cerebellar peduncles look like large, thick commas on either side, per Nauta (1986), but they're buried in other (middle cerebellar) peduncular or deep cerebellar white matter.

    1a. By the way, **olivocerebellar fibers** constitute the largest component of inferior cerebellar peduncle (Carpenter and Sutin, 1983).

2. **Via** (left) **inferior cerebellar peduncle**, axons pass, now as climbing fibers, to (left) **cerebellar hemisphere** in the case of (right) principal nucleus of the inferior olive, specifically to the **Purkinje cell layer.**

3. If we consider other inferior olivary subnuclei, their axons arrive at other cerebellar/Purkinje-cell-layer destinations (e.g., **medial accessory olive** to *flocculus* and *vermis*; you might be interested to know that the medial accessory olive is especially developed in the sonar-savvy porpoise, compared to humans [Baizer et al., 2011]).

*

What's dorsal to **medial lemniscus** above my head? Moving ventral to dorsal, we've identified these structures previously:

> **central tegmental tract,** a bit lateral to the medial lemnisci, ends in medulla as the *amiculum* **of the inferior olive;**

> **tectospinal tract,** which retains its intimate proximity to medial longitudinal fasciculus, then:

> **medial longitudinal fasciculus.**

We're quite not done. At our axial level, dorsal to the medial longitudinal fasciculus, are nuclei just under the floor of the fourth ventricle on either side of the midline seam. Their location tempts one to think of some motor function akin to other, very midline nuclei (think CN IV nuclei for example), but what *are* they?

*

> **RULE #8**: If you're in medulla, and if you see midline nuclei just ventral to the floor of the fourth ventricle, then DON'T assume that you've found the hypoglossal nuclei.

*

Maybe we could call them nuclei *presiding* over the hypoglossal nuclei, since we're now above/higher than the level of the hypoglossal (CN XII) nuclei. So be it, since the same thought occurred to anatomists a long time ago, but let's use Latin.

The vertical distance between CN VI nuclei and CN XII nuclei is filled by the column-shaped ***nucleus prepositus hypoglossi*** on either side of the midline (McCrea and Horn, 2006). It's a nucleus of interneurons; it's involved in the control of eye movements probably *not* by way of projections into near-by medial longitudinal fasciculus (McCrea and Baker, 1985).[9] Its interneurons connect to and/or from many nodes, among them: vestibular nuclei, paramedian pontine reticular formation, inferior olive, *flocculus*, *nodulus*, *vermis*, superior colliculus, thalamus, and extraocular motor nuclei. I have abbreviated the list; there are other start and end points related to this curiously central structure.

---

[9] We should probably disabuse ourselves of the notion that the medial longitudinal fasciculus is the only avenue that connects vestibular nuclei to ocular motor nuclei. The connections of the *nucleus prepositus hypoglossi* are an example, as is the **ascending tract of Deiters**, which is an excitatory pathway from medial vestibular nucleus to CN III nucleus. Without crossing the midline, it ascends lateral to the medial longitudinal fasciculus.

39

Oblivious to Ocular Lateropulsion

Some years ago, residents in our program asked whether I could review a few years of Residency In-Training Examinations, distill all prior questions related to neuroanatomy, then give a talk about what trainees needed to know for the next exam. At least they were honest about what they wanted.

In prepping for the lecture, I ran across the term *ocular lateropulsion*. Taking a break from axial sections, I'll ask now: what is it?

1. Let's start with normality. Open both eyes, look straight ahead, perhaps at some distant object directly in front of you. Now close your eyes for a few seconds. Now, open them. Are your eyes still fixed on the object? If yes, then we'll call that normal.

2. Now consider the phenomenon. The patient seems relaxed, as relaxed as one can be while being examined. You instruct her to look straight ahead.

What if her eyes don't look, to you, exactly straight ahead? You're not sure, but it seems as if she's gazing at something off to one side. The deviation could be subtle; it could be obvious.

I'm not discussing anything like a skew deviation or anything else but a sense that the eyes don't quite look straight ahead.[10]

3. You ask her, "are you looking straight ahead?" She says, "yup."

4. We'll have her close her eyes for a few seconds. In that interval, her eyes conjugately roam to one side in the horizontal plane. We know, because when she opens her eyes, they are deviated incompletely or very completely to one side. Regardless, they have moved without question, lateropulsed.

In a series of 14 consecutive cases reported in 1974 (all with ocular lateropulsion), we read:

> The lateral deviation in all cases appeared when the patients were requested to relax and "gaze straight ahead." *All* patients were quite unaware of the lateral deviation (with the exception of one . . . [whose eyes "were locked" to the right side]); to reach the mid-position of the eyes they had voluntarily to deviate the eyes in the opposite direction. Some patients, however, were not able to maintain *a* position of steady, voluntary straight-forward or contralateral gaze. In six patients . . . the tonic pull could be overcome only for *a* very short while. When they were requested to keep the gaze in a direction opposite to the conjugate deviation, the eyes slowly drifted away to the tonically deviated position. The drift was characteristically smooth "*as* if the eyeballs were pulled by elastic bands"; it was occasionally interrupted by rapid and large nystagmoid beats in the direction of attempted

---

10   Lateropulsion and skew deviation aren't mutually exclusive. Regarding the latter, the following is useful: "In typical skew deviations, the higher eye is contralateral to a medullary lesion and ipsilateral to a mid pontine (the level at which otolith projections decussate the brainstem) or midbrain lesion. . . . in the case of a left lateral medullary syndrome, an ocular tilt reaction might involve left head tilt, right hyperdeviation, and countertroll of the eyes (upper poles) toward the left shoulder . . ." (Frohman et al., 2008). But in my vignette, I'm interested in a clue that lateropulsion will occur when fixation is lost–i.e., when she closes her eyes.

voluntary gaze . . . [emphases are original to the paper] (Hörnsten, 1974b).

The above is worth parsing. Why? Because there's relevance especially to the medulla. Also because, if we don't read the passage with care, we'll miss something stunning.

The 14 cases weren't instances of a conjugate gaze palsy. They *were* able to get the eyes past the midline . . . in the direction opposite to the lateropulsion. It might have been effortful, but still possible: some weren't able to maintain *a* position of steady, voluntary straight-forward or contralateral gaze; or, the elastic-band pull could be overcome only briefly; but conjugate gaze to the side opposite the lateropulsion was doable.

Why were *all* patients, save the one whose eyes *locked* to one side, "quite unaware of the lateral deviation"? They were unaware or oblivious, because, from their point of view, they looked straight ahead.

Is there a sense in which the idea of *what's straight ahead* changes?

By the way, the 14 cases were all medullary infarctions. As a rule of thumb, the direction of lateropulsion pointed to the side of the lesion.

*

Let's experiment on our normal selves again.
1. There's a tree with a big trunk in a nearby park. It stands alone without anything around it. The trunk is tilted a bit against the snowy ground of winter.
2. We wonder if it's possible to make the trunk look straight up and down. It tilts to the right, maybe by 10 degrees.
3. We tilt our head about 10 degrees to our right; does that make the trunk straight? I tried it. My answer is: I can sorta make it look straight, but I know it's not. How do I know?
4. We recall from physics that, assuming a mass isn't influenced by other masses, it falls in a plumb vertical line in a gravitational field.
5. How do I know the vertical line in the gravitational field in the park? It's actually that vertical line which allows me to conclude that the tree trunk tilts in space. The tilt is relative to the verticality. Tilting my head doesn't help.
6. There's an objective vertical which generally matches what has been called the subjective visual vertical.

Quoting again from the series of 14 cases, *"Torsion of the visual fields* [author's emphasis] was initially experienced by three patients . . .. This phenomenon was very dramatic in [two] patients, who felt as if the surroundings were tilted 180° for the first few minutes. A 90° tilt persisted in [one] patient for several days" (Hörnsten, 1974a). A subjective visual vertical at odds with the objective vertical as determined by gravity occurs in brainstem pathology, particular medullary pathology (Dieterich and Brandt, 1993).

For completeness, we should note that some argue that paroxysmal tilts of the world as we view it differ from actual measurements of the subjective visual vertical:

> . . . a pathologic "tilt illusion," in which the world is seen to be on its side or inverted, is experienced transiently by patients with lateral medullary, thalamic, or even cerebral infarct or hemorrhage. However, central or peripheral lesions typically do not cause complaints of an abnormal sense of the vertical, and any disturbance goes undetected unless patients are tested when deprived of visual information [they are tested in darkness] (Sharpe, 2003).

Lack of detection is my interest in the passage. You can't *not* detect a sensation of environment tilt: up becomes down and vice versa. And there are variations—90° tilts, etc.—in reported series (Sierra-Hidalgo et al., 2012). Yet, ever so subtly and without personal awareness, a sense of what's straight ahead and of gravity's true axis can change in a medullary process.

Subjective perception sounds redundant (what perception isn't?), but we actively discriminate between the ways or means to achieve it:

> A scheme of 'orientation in space' can be mediated relatively independently by visual, vestibular or proprioceptive channels.. . . the subject can experience the co-existence of contradicting perceptions. When pushed to make a realistic appraisal of his orientation, the sensory channel(s) which, from experience, appear more veridical, are selected for the task.

I wish the authors had used a different word than "veridical," which one can easily misread as "vertical." The point is clear nevertheless: we know down and up by vision, vestibular function, and by haptic sense or proprioception. If we require a realistic appraisal of the environment, we determine what seems true based on some kind of recalibration or reweighting:

> . . . such re-weighting may be a requisite underlying compensation for the postural and perceptual effects of acute balance disorders . . ..

Sounds like a plan. But what about environmental tilts in which something's very obviously non-veridical in perception?

> This [re-weighting] scheme, however, may not apply to acute, focal brainstem lesions with marked lateropulsion, e.g. lateral medullary syndrome. In this case a tighter association between motor and perceptual aspects may exist, but only the SVV [subjective visual vertical], not the SPV [subjective postural vertical], has been measured in such patients. However . . . studies of the visual vertical are not necessarily representative of other aspects of spatial orientation (Bisdorff et al., 1996).

I realize that I conflate thoughts about lateropulsion and sensations of environmental tilt. My rationale for doing so is to illuminate how awry the world can look in the context of lateral medullary disease. The lateral medulla, by the way, is where proprioceptive (leminiscal) and oculovestibular fibers are in intimate proximity. Consider the plain difficulty experienced by the one patient aware of his extreme lateropulsion–the one whose eyes locked to the right:

> The patient constantly preferred to keep his head turned to the left. In this way the eyes were kept in dextroversion when he looked at objects in front of him. He complained of a sensation of "locking the eyes" to the right, and attempted gaze to the left produced a definite feeling of discomfort which was difficult to verbalize distinctly. An

increased sensation of instability of the visual field seemed to be a dominant feature (Hörnsten, 1974b).

Perhaps instability of the visual field reaches an apogee in cases of torsion of those fields.

*

If the subjective differs the from objective in any axis aside from vertical, a person wouldn't necessarily acknowledge any difference to herself, absent some frame of reference *like* the gravitational vertical.

Hence the response "yup" to the woman whose eyes look subtly and conjugately askance from our examiner's vantage point?

The last sentence is meant to be a question, which you can cogitate at your leisure.

*

To come full circle, I recall that the answer book for the Residency In-Training Examination talked about how ocular lateropulsion in a lateral medullary syndrome is likely due to a lesion of olivocerebellar climbing fibers. I've since lost that book, which didn't reference the statement, if memory serves.

Maybe there are other answers aside from *a* lesion of olivocerebellar climbing fibers. What about a lesion of vestibular nuclei or of their many efferents in medulla or even in pons? Unless you're the patient herself, it's hard to be oblivious to ocular lateropulsion. The phenomenon begs questions about how we unconsciously represent the world relative to our own position and orientation in space.

40

Canonical Medulla

By canonical, I mean an axial section of medulla in which we visualize all of the following together (in alphabetical order):

Ambiguus nucleus (related to CN IX and X),
Anterolateral fasciculus (a.k.a. spinothalamic tract),
Cochlear nuclei (CN VIII),

Descending tract and nucleus of CN V (a.k.a. spinal tract and nucleus of CN V),

Dorsal motor nucleus of Vagus (CN X),
Hypoglossal nucleus (CN XII),

Inferior cerebellar peduncle (a.k.a. restiform body–note that at our current level we visualize nothing of the *brachium pontis* or *brachium conjunctivum*; in other words, we are well caudal to the middle and superior cerebellar peduncles),

Inferior olive,
Medial lemniscus,
Medial longitudinal fasciculus,
Pyramid,
Solitary nucleus and tract (related to CN's VII, IX, and X),

Tectospinal tract, and
Vestibular nuclear column (CN VIII).

We've encountered the boldfaced items in this seminar. At the current level, it's relatively easy to organize the nuclei which we *haven't* yet visualized.

Applying a principle from neural development, we divide into alar/dorsal and basal/ventral based on sensory and motor nuclei, respectively. Where's the demarcation between alar/dorsal/sensory and basal/ventral/motor in medulla?

*

We require just two points to determine a line. I'll choose two that are noticeable: descending or spinal nucleus of CN V, which we've met in rostral cuts, and solitary nucleus and tract (associated with CN's VII, IX, X), which is new to us. Solitary nucleus is hard to miss in atlases. Like the descending nucleus of CN V, solitary nucleus is located in the lateral medulla.

Draw a line along the under/ventral sides of spinal nucleus and of solitary nucleus. Extrapolate it towards the floor of the fourth ventricle. The line points you directly at the *sulcus limitans* of Wilhelm His, Sr.

The *sulcus limitans* indents the fourth-ventricular floor just medial to the **vestibular triangle**. As we recall, the vestibular nuclei comprise a column that's present from medulla into pons, always lateral in its location in brainstem.

*

Nuclei derived from basal plate, **medial to the line**, including the **dorsal motor nucleus of Vagus** (CN X) and the **hypoglossal nucleus** (CN XII), are *motor.*

Nucleus ambiguus (related to CN IX and X) isn't easily seen in atlases, but its neurons are not ambiguously located. They're motor to soft palate, pharynx, and larynx. They're all medial to the line and dorsal to the principal nucleus of inferior olive.

If we move caudally towards the cervicomedullary junction, motor neurons contributing to the **spinal accessory nerve (CN XI)** are also medial to the line.

*

Nuclei derived from alar plate, **lateral to the line**, including the **solitary nucleus** and **sensory nucleus of CN V** themselves, the **vestibular nuclei** in the vestibular triangle, and **cochlear nuclei**, which drape themselves over the lateral aspect of the inferior cerebellar peduncles on either side, are *sensory*.

The solitary nucleus and tract receive fibers from CN's VII, IX, and X, related to taste (anterior 2/3 and posterior 1/3 of tongue) and visceral sensation from the heart, lungs, and gut.

Some facial sensory fibers (pinna and tragus of the ear) from CN VII and CN IX contribute to sensory nucleus and tract of CN V.

If we move caudally towards the cervicomedullary junction, sensory nuclei, such as the **gracile and cuneate nuclei**, are lateral to the line.

*

We're almost done, but strap in for the last mile or so of travel.

Teachers win points with students by way of their memory games. For the brainstem *as a whole*, for example (Gates, 2011), consider these four rules, all conveniently related to the number 4:

There are *four* structures in the midline starting with the letter M [Motor/corticospinal/pyramidal pathway, Medial lemsisci, Motor nuclei, Medial longitudinal fasciculus].

There are *four* structures in the lateral brainstem starting with the letter S [Spinothalamic pathway, Sympathetic pathway, Sensory nucleus of the fifth cranial nerve, Spinocerebellar Tract].

The lower *four* cranial nerves are in the medulla, the middle *four* are in the pons, and the first *four* cranial nerves are above the pons, with the third and fourth in the midbrain.

The *four* motor cranial nerves that are in the midline are the four that divide evenly into 12 (except for 1 and 2)– that is, 3, 4, 6, and 12.

Two structures mentioned above have escaped discussion in this seminar: the Sympathetic pathway and Spinocerebellar tract. We won't ignore them, but we should acknowledge that they're tricky in anatomical terms. I've always enjoyed mnemonics of the sort just quoted, but my reason for liking them has changed over time. Today, for example, the riff on the number four makes me think harder about the actual anatomy.

There are two spinocerebellar tracts, first, a dorsal or posterior tract that feeds into inferior cerebellar peduncle without decussation across the midline. One doesn't see dorsal spinocerebellar tract above the medulla. Second, there's a ventral or anterior tract that can be found at all levels of lateral brainstem, but its route is roundabout. As with the dorsal tract, information transmitted has to do with unconscious proprioception (e.g., afferents from Golgi tendon organs in the limbs); decussation across the midline happens segmentally in spinal cord–for illustration, from right hemicord across to left–, then the tract ascends in the left lateral funiculus of cord, then lateral to (left) inferior olive in medulla, then lateral to the horizontally oriented (left) medial leminscus in pons, then lateral to the (left) superior cerebellar peduncle at the pontomesencephalic border; fibers then cross the midline (they cross once again, now towards the right) in the decussation of the superior cerebellar peduncles en route to cerebellum. Is dorsal spinocerebellar tract lateral in medulla? Yes, only in medulla. Is ventral spinocerebellar tract lateral in medulla, pons, and midbrain? Nominally yes, but the second rule of 4 primarily addresses features of a lateral medullary syndrome.

Previously, we mentioned but didn't fully discuss the sympathetic pathway within brainstem. I'll cut and paste to aid memory:

> . . . hypothalamic axons also descend in the **dorsal tegmental pathway**, although there's debate over whether, for example, projections from parvocelluluar paraventricular nucleus of hypothalamus connect monosynaptically with neurons in the spinal cord's intermediolateral grey column, from whence second-order arise in the sympathetic pupillodilatory pathway.

Dorsal tegmentum in low midbrain–tegmentum there is ventral to tectum, if you recall–refers us to the vicinity of CN IV (trochlear) nuclei, which stare at us a last time. First-order neurons in the sympathetic pathway aren't always lateral as they are in medulla. One way not to forget that anatomy is to think about a syndrome familiar to neuroophthalmologists: "The combination of an ipsilateral Horner syndrome (first-order) and contralateral superior oblique palsy suggests a lesion of the trochlear nucleus of its fascicle in the brainstem" (Biousse and Newman, 2009). I trust that one understands why the palsy is contralateral to the lesion. One might also expect a head tilt towards the side of the superior oblique palsy, but the miosis/ptosis is on the same side as the low, paramedian mesencephalic lesion.

The first and second rules related to the number 4 address, for all intents and purposes, the demarcation between basal and alar plates best seen in the medulla. Those who teach about the *sulcus limitans* and the division of basal from alar, however, must confess what Nieuwenhuys himself called a limitation irrespective of overall explanatory power. We need look no further than the inferior olive to be humbled.

The nucleus is of *alar plate origin*. So why is it medial to the line marked by our three landmarks (*sulcus limitans* at the floor of the fourth ventricle, the ventral side of solitary nucleus, the ventral side of spinal nucleus of CN V)?

Think even about the pons, where there is no inferior olive: pontine nuclei . . . are also of *alar plate origin*. So why are those alar entities, all those nuclei, so prominently located in the *basis pontis*?

The short answer is that the locations of inferior olive and pontine nuclei in adult human neuroanatomy are the consequence of lateral-to-medial tangential migrations during development.

Nieuwenhuys' work over many years, summarized in his 2011 paper, has informed this seminar from the start. As we end our tour, it seems there's new work to be done:

> . . . topological maps, derived from the brainstems of adult specimens, have certain important limitations, irrespective of their overall explanatory power. The exceptions discussed [e.g., inferior olive, pontine nuclei] make plain that the topological procedure does not project all cell masses back to their sites of origin and therewith to their primary topological positions. Conversely, it is now clear that the preparation of a *topological supermap*, showing the genuine primary positions of all constituent nuclei in

the brainstem of a given species, would require extensive neuroembryological studies, involving, *inter alia*, the expression patterns of numerous developmental regulatory genes and the tracing of all tangential migrations.

A supermap? We'll stop quite shy of that.

41

A Note on Brainstem Vasculature

From a 1961 paper, we read: "In a study of this type it is not sufficient merely to determine which of the large arteries is occluded–although previous authors have gone no further. A more exact delineation of the pattern of arterial distribution to the infarcted territory is necessary . . . " (Fisher et al., 1961). For 50 or so pages, he and his coauthors discuss vascular pathology affecting the lateral medulla. After a review of prior literature that starts the paper, they opine, "It would appear from this summary of the literature that the term 'posterior inferior cerebellar artery syndrome' was from the beginning a misnomer." Then the writing starts in earnest–a report of 16 cases of lateral medullary infarction, 14 of which had vascular occlusions, 12 of which had vertebral occlusions, and only 2 of which had occlusions of the posterior inferior cerebellar artery.

Many years ago, I had one encounter–my only contact, by phone–with the lead author. I had the sense that his was a medical intellect compared to which all others had proven merely insufficient. With the ghost of him in my ear, what does one dare say about arteries to the entire brainstem? Like the approach throughout this seminar, I only offer aspects that have interested or helped me over time–all in the hope that the writing helps you, too.

As routine textbook chapters attest (Miyawaki, 2014), humans have the same larger arteries in the posterior circulation: vertebrals, basilar, superior cerebellar(s), and posterior cerebral(s). Vascular variability has to do with nuances regarding those large vessels as well as with the arteries of smaller caliber associated with them. For example, if the vertebrals aren't of the same caliber, then which is typically larger (the left one, perhaps)? If the left vertebral is larger, does the basilar tend to bend one way rather than the other (to the right, perhaps)? The anterior spinal artery is said to arise from both vertebrals, but where the two vertebrals fuse into the basilar is variable, so the level where the anterior spinal artery arises is also variable (Carpenter and Sutin, 1983). The origin the posterior inferior cerebellar artery is typically the vertebral, but proximal basilar is a variant; if the origin is the vertebral, sometimes the take-off of posterior inferior cerebellar artery is extradural, sometimes intradural. Not everyone has two anterior, inferior cerebellar arteries . . ..

Anatomical nuances are legion.

The reason why patterns of arterial distribution to an infarcted territory are important has to do with an inescapable fact that there's variation in the territories supplied by any given vessel, whether of larger or smaller caliber. And there's much overlap between arterial areas.

With the above in mind, and with preemptive apology to those of more encyclopedic bias, one can summarize the paramedian and circumferential supply of the brainstem at representative levels. The wedge-shaped approximate areas per axial level have indistinct or variable borders between them:

> In the hemi-medulla, from midline to lateral: territories of the **anterior spinal, vertebral,** and **posterior inferior cerebellar arteries;**

> In the mid-/hemi-pons, roughly at the level of the facial colliculi, from midline to lateral: territories of the **basilar** and **anterior inferior cerebellar arteries;**

> In the upper hemi-pons, from midline to lateral: territories of the **basilar** and **superior cerebellar arteries.**

> In the hemi-midbrain, from midline to lateral: territories of the **basilar** and **posterior cerebral arteries.**

Unilateral ischemic lesions abutting the midline seem reliably to obey it.

*

I'll conclude with case 5 from the 1961 series.

A 70 year-old woman had had problems with high blood pressure for three years prior to her presentation. Blood pressures ran roughly 190/100. Her only hypertensive symptom was occasional dizziness, about which we know little.

Six days prior to admission she experienced brief bouts of weakness and dizziness.

Five days prior, she had a particularly severe attack in which she experienced a spinning sensation. Her whole head hurt; she thought her left eye was out of focus.

Four days prior, she was "up and about," but still felt dizzy with a generalized headache. That afternoon, she found it difficult to swallow. She had double vision.

Three days prior, she felt an intense numbness of her right face. One of her legs felt weak.

Two days prior, she occasionally saw objects upside down. She continued to have problems swallowing. She felt restless.

By the time she presented to hospital, difficulty handling oral secretions had worsened; she often choked. Her speech was thick, with progression to speechlessness. She felt whole-body weakness.

On examination, she was febrile to 103° Fahrenheit and tachycardic (100 beats per minute). Blood pressure was 170/80 mmHg. Respirations were 15 per minute. She was cooperative, but unable to speak. Her pupils were small bilaterally, but both reacted to light and accommodation. There was nystagmus on upgaze, questionably so on lateral gaze. Sensation was diminished over the right face. Corneal reflexes were absent bilaterally. She had a left CN VI nerve palsy. She could not swallow. The tongue protruded weakly in the midline. She had a flaccid right hemiplegia. The left arm and leg moved slightly. Deep tendon reflexes were trace in the arms, save for a slightly greater right biceps reflex compared to the left. Knee and ankle jerks were absent. Both toes were extensor.

Her respirations slowed to 5 per minute. Stupor followed. She died on the second house day (Fisher et al., 1961, case 5).

*

The pace of the story, never mind the ending, disturbs.

Since we know that all 16 cases of the series involved infarction of the lateral medulla, questions arise.

1. When did hers occur?
2. On day 5 prior to admission, what's to be made of her left eye being out of focus? Do we discard the information, because it's monocular? Answer: we could, but the series referenced in chapter 39 (Hörnsten, 1974a, 1974b) describes such monocular symptoms. Why, then, the left eye?
3. Did hers occur when the swallowing difficulty commenced (4 days prior to admission)?
4. On day 3 prior to admission, does the addition of the right face numbness cinch a medullary localization? If so, what's to be made of the weakness in one of her legs?
5. If you discount the weakness on day 3, then what's to be made of the flaccid right hemiplegia in her examination on the day of admission?
6. Two days prior, when she occasionally saw the world upside down, was that when her stroke happened or were the sensations of environmental tilt epiphenomena?
7. In the reported examination, why were both pupils small and why were corneal reflexes absent *bilaterally*?
8. Regarding the left CN VI palsy, if the lesion were nuclear, we'd rather expect a left facial palsy and an associate conjugate gaze palsy (to the left), but we see neither.
9. If you invoke a lesion of left paramedian pontine reticular formation, how does the exam not corroborate your thought? Answer: if paramedian pontine reticular formation, wouldn't you expect a conjugate gaze palsy to the left (*both* eyes unable to look leftward)?
10. Why were both toes extensor?
11. Why the stupor?

You're eager for answers. I understand.

Recall, though, that the motivation for this third seminar was to get you to think like a local for yourself. The authors themselves don't rush in with answers to the 11 or even more questions that you could ask about the 70 year-old woman:

> This case is an example of the lateral medullary syndrome associated with thrombosis of the right VA [vertebral artery], and accompanied by a separate pontine infarct. [On review of the pathology,] [t]he lateral medullary infarct at the mid-olivary level accounted for most of the patient's prodromal and early manifestations. The vessel of supply to the region of the medullary infarct was identified as a branch of the VA [vertebral artery]. This case illustrates that the [lateral medullary] syndrome is not always benign, but can presage a basilar artery thrombosis if the involved VA [vertebral artery] is the only adequate source of supply to the basilar territory. Damage to the brainstem was likely more extensive than portrayed in the stained [pathological] section since the pontine lesion could not have accounted for the stupor or the 6th nerve palsy (Fisher et al., 1961).

Welcome to an honest case in which you have to think *through* your fundamental three choices. The brainstem, healthy or not, will be found in your clinical examination.

REFERENCES, BY SEMINAR, FOR VOLUME ONE

References for the First Seminar

General Neuroanatomy:

Brodal, A. *Neurological Anatomy in Relation to Clinical Medicine*. Third ed. New York/Oxford: Oxford University Press, 1981.

Carpenter, Malcolm B. and Sutin, Jerome. *Human Neuroanatomy*. Eighth ed. Baltimore/London: Williams and Wilkins, 1983.

Nieuwenhuys R., Voogd J., van Huijzen C. *The Human Central Nervous System*. Fourth ed. Berlin/Heidelberg/New York: Springer Verlag, 2008.

Other Books:

Hebb, D.O. *Essay on Mind*. New York: Psychology Press, 2009.

Hubel, David H. *Eye, Brain, and Vision*. New York: Scientific American Library, 1995.

Langman, Jan. *Medical Embryology*. Fourth ed. Baltimore: Williams and Wilkins, 1981.

Newton, Isaac [Sir]. *Opticks or A Treatise of the Reflections, Refractions, Inflections, & Colours of Light* [based on the fourth edition, London 1730]. New York: Dover, 1979.

Swanson, Larry W. *Brain Architecture. Understanding the Basic Plan.* Second ed. New York: Oxford University Press, 2012.

Volpe, Joseph J. *Neurology of the Newborn.* Second ed. Philadelphia: W.B. Saunders, 1987.

*

Articles:

Alvarez-Bolado G, Rosenfeld MG, Swanson LW. Model of forebrain regionalization based on spatiotemporal patterns of POU-III homeobox gene expression, birthdates, and morphological features. *Journal of Comparative Neurology* 1995;355:237-295.

Anonymous. Cerebral localisation. *British Medical Journal* 1877;2:699.

Bender M. Brain control of conjugate horizontal and vertical eye movements. A survey of the structural and functional correlates. *Brain* 1980:103;23-69.

Chisholm A, Tessier-Lavigne M. Conservation and divergence of axon guidance mechanisms. *Current Opinion in Neurobiology* 1999;9:603-615.

Collett T. Stereopsis in toads. *Nature* 1977;267:349-351.

Crelin ES, Netter FH, Shapter RK. Development of the nervous system. A logical approach to neuroanatomy. *Clinical Symposia* 1974;26(2), reprinted as a monograph, Summit, NJ: Ciba-Geigy, 1974.

Davidoff RA. The pyramidal tract. *Neurology* 1990;40:332-339.

De Lussanet MHE, Osse JWM. An ancestral twist explains the contralateral forebrain and the optic chiasm in vertebrates. *Animal Biology* 2012;62:193-216.

Dickson BJ. Molecular mechanisms of axon guidance. *Science* 2002;298:1959-1964.

Dickson BJ, Zou Y. Navigating intermediate targets: the nervous system midline. *Cold Spring Harbor Perspectives in Biology* 2010;2:a002055.

Echelard Y, Epstein DJ, St-Jacques B, Shen L, Mohler J, McMahon JA, McMahon AP. Sonic hedgehog, a member of a family of putative signaling molecules, is implicated in the regulation of CNS polarity. *Cell* 1993;75:1417-1430.

Ferland RJ, Eyaid W, Collura RV, Tully LD, Hill RS, Al-Nouri D, Al-Rumayan A, Topcu M, Gascon G, Bodell A, Shugart YY, Ruvolo M, Walsh CA. Abnormal cerebellar development and axonal decussation due to mutations in *AHI1* in Joubert syndrome. *Nature Genetics* 2004;36:1008-1013.

Florence SL, Wall JT, Kaas JH. Somatotopic organization of inputs from the hand to the spinal gray and cuneate nucleus of monkeys with observations on the cuneate nucleus of humans. *Journal of Comparative Neurology* 1989;286:48-70.

Gilles FH. Myelination in the neonatal brain. *Human Pathology* 1976;7:244-248.

Hikosaka O. The habenula: from stress evasion to value-based decision-making. *Nature Reviews/Neuroscience* 2010;11:503-513.

Horn AKE, Leigh RJ. The anatomy and physiology of the ocular motor system. *Handbook of Clinical Neurology, Neuro-ophthalmology* (Third Series) 2011;102:21-69.

Jeffery G. Architecture of the optic chiasm and the mechanisms that sculpt its development. *Physiological Reviews* 2001;81:1393-1414.

Joubert M, Eisenring JJ, Robb JP, Andermann F. Familial agenesis of the cerebellar vermis. A syndrome of episodic hyperpnea, abnormal eye movements, and retardation. *Neurology* 1969;19:813-825.

Kinsbourne M. Somatic twist: a model for the evolution of decussation. *Neuropsychology* 2013;27:511-515.

Lumsden AGS, Davies AM. Earliest sensory nerve fibres are guided to peripheral targets by attractants other than nerve growth factor. *Nature* 1983;306:786-788.

Lumsden A, Krumlauf R. Patterning the vertebrate neuraxis. *Science* 1996;274:1109-1115.

Mueller F, O'Rahilly R. The first appearance of the future cerebral hemispheres in the human embryo at stage 14. *Anatomy and Embryology* 1988;177:495-511.

Nanni L, Ming JE, Bocian M, Steinhaus K, Bianchi DW, de Die-Dmulders C, Giannotti A, Imaizumi K, Jones KL, Del Campo M, Martin RA, Meinecke P, Pierpont MEM, Robin NH, Young ID, Roessler E, Muenke M. The mutational spectrum of the Sonic Hedgehog gene in holoprosencephaly: SHH mutations cause a significant proportion of autosomal dominant holoprosencephaly. *Human Molecular Genetics* 1999;8:2479-2488.

Nieuwenhuys R. The structural, functional, and molecular organization of the brainstem. *Frontiers in Neuroanatomy* 2011;5:33. doi: 10.3389/fnana.2011.00033.

Sarnat HB, Netsky MG. When does a ganglion become a brain? Evolutionary origin of the central nervous system. *Seminars in Pediatric Neurology* 2002;9:240-253.

Shinbrot T, Young W. Why decussate? Topological constraints on 3D wiring. *The Anatomical Record* 2008;291:1278-1292.

Sperry RW. Cerebral organization and behavior. *Science* 1961;133:1749-1757.

Stoeckli ET. Understand axon guidance: are we nearly there yet? *Development* 2018;145, dev 151415, doi:10.1242/dev.151415.

Vulliemoz S, Raineteau O, Jabaudon D. Reaching beyond the midline: why are human brains cross wired? *Lancet Neurology* 2005;4:87-99.

Wadsworth WG, Hedgecock EM. Hierarchical guidance cues in the developing nervous system of C. elegans. *BioEssays* 1996;18:355-362.

Yachnis AT, Rorke LB. Neuropathology of Joubert syndrome. *Journal of Child Neurology* 1999;14:655-659.

References for the Second Seminar

Books:

Aminoff, Michael J. *Brown-Séquard. A Visionary of Science*. New York: Raven Press, 1993.

Brodmann, Korbinian. *Brodmann's Localisation in the Cerebral Cortex*. [trans. Garey, LJ] New York: Springer, 2006

Carpenter, Malcolm B. and Sutin, Jerome. *Human Neuroanatomy*. [8th ed.] Baltimore and London: Williams and Wilkins, 1983.

Deacon, Terrence W. *The Symbolic Species. The Co-evolution of Language and the Brain*. New York and London: W.W. Norton, 1997.

Dehaene, Stanislas. *Reading in the Brain. The Science and Evolution of a Human Invention*. New York: Viking, 2009

Eggert, Gertrude H. *Wernicke's Works on Aphasia: A Sourcebook and Review*. The Hague: Mouton, 1977.

Farah, Martha J. *Visual Agnosia. Disorders of Object Recognition and What They Tell Us about Normal Vision*. Cambridge and London: MIT Press, 1990.

Finger, Stanley. *Origins of Neuroscience. A History of Explorations into Brain Function*. Oxford and New York: Oxford, 1994.

Finger, Stanley. *Minds Behind the Brain: A History of the Pioneers and their Discoveries*. New York: Oxford, 2000.

Geschwind, Norman. *Selected Papers on Language and the Brain: Boston Studies in the Philosophy of Science* (vol. XVI), eds. Cohen, Robert S. and Wartofsky, Marx W. Dordrecht and Boston: D. Reidel Publishing, 1974.

Goodglass, Harold and Kaplan, Edith. *The Assessment of Aphasia and Related Disorders*. [2nd ed.] Philadelphia: Lea and Febiger, 1983.

Havelock, Eric A. *The Literate Revolution in Greece and Its Cultural Consequences*. Princeton: Princeton University Press, 1982.

Haymaker, Webb and Baer, Karl A., eds. *Founders of Neurology: One Hundred and Thirty-Three Biographical Sketches*. Springfield: Charles C. Thomas, 1953.

Hunt, Morton. *The Story of Psychology*. New York: Anchor, 1994.

Kahle, Werner. *Nervous System and Sensory Organs*. [3rd revised edition, trans. H.L. and A.D. Dayan, Volume 3 of Kahle W., Leonhardt H, Platzer W. *Color Atlas and Textbook of Human Anatomy*] Stuttgart and New York: Georg Thieme, 1986.

Lidwell, William, Holden, Kritina, and Butler, Jill. *Universal Principles of Design*. Beverly, MA: Rockport, 2010. (The book as a whole is of interest, but I allude particularly to the chapter entitled "Structural Forms.")

Locke, Simeon. *Mind. An Emergent Property*. Bloomington: Xlibris, 2014.

Luria, A.R. *Human Brain and Psychological Processes*. [trans. Haigh, B.] New York and London: Harper and Row, 1966.

Luria, A.R. *The Man with a Shattered World. The History of a Brain Wound*. [trans. Solotaroff, L.] Cambridge: Harvard University Press, 1972.

Luria, A.R. *The Working Brain. An Introduction of Neuropsychology*. [trans. Haigh, B.] New York: Basic Books, 1973.

Luria, Aleksandr Romanovich. *Higher Cortical Functions in Man*. [2nd ed., trans. Haigh, B.] New York: Basic Books, 1980.

McHenry, Lawrence C., Jr. *Garrison's History of Neurology*. Springfield: Charles C. Thomas, 1969.

Mesulam M.-Marsel. *Principles of Behavioral and Cognitive Neurology*. [2nd ed.] Oxford and New York: Oxford, 2000.

Nolte, John. *The Human Brain. An Introduction to Its Functional Anatomy*. [4th ed.] St. Louis: Mosby, 1999.

Shepherd, Gordon M [ed.] *The Synaptic Organization of the Brain*. [4th ed.] New York and Oxford: Oxford University Press, 1998.

Wernicke C. *Der Aphasische Symptomencomplex: Eine Psychologische Studie auf Anatomische Basis*. Breslau: Cohn, 1874. [I translated the original text and checked myself using Eggert, 1977 and the translation referenced as Wernicke, 1969.]

*

Articles and Chapters in Books:

Anonymous. The University of Vienna, *British Medical Journal* 1874;2(713):282-283.

Anonymous. An introduction to the life and work of John Hughlings Jackson. *Medical History Supplement* 2007; (26): 3–34.

Bellugi U, Lichtenberger L, Jones W, Lai Z, St. George M. The neurocognitive profile of Williams syndrome: a complex pattern of strengths and weaknesses. *Journal of Cognitive Neuroscience* 2000;12 supplement 1:7-29.

Berker EA, Berker AT, Smith A. Translation of Broca's 1865 report: localization of speech in the third left frontal convolution. *Archives of Neurology* 1986;43:1065-1072.

Bernal B, Ardila A. The role of the arcuate fasciculus in conduction aphasia. *Brain* 2009;132:2309-2316.

Beuren AJ, Apitz J, Harmjanz D. Supravalvular aortic stenosis in association with mental retardation and a certain facial appearance. *Circulation* 1962;26:1235-1240.

Braga RM, Buckner RL. Parallel interdigitated distributed networks within the individual estimated by intrinsic functional connectivity. *Neuron* 2017;95:457-471.

Broca P. Perte de la parole, ramollisement chronique et destruction partielle du lobe antérieur gauche du cerveau [Loss of speech, chronic softening and partial destruction of the left anterior lobe of the brain]. *Bulletins de la Société d'Anthropologie* 1861a;2:235-238, available in translation in Wilkins, Robert H (ed.). *Neurosurgical Classics.* American Association of Neurological Surgeons, 1992, pp. 63-64.

Broca P. Remarks on the seat of the faculty of articulated language, following an observation of aphemia (loss of speech). *Bulletin de la Société Anatomique* 1861b;6:330-357, in translation by Christopher D. Green at http://psychclassics.yorku.ca/Broca/aphemie-e.htm.

Catani M, ffytche DH. The rises and falls of disconnection syndromes. *Brain* 2005;128:2224-2239.

Catani M, Mesulam M. The arcuate fasciculus and the disconnection theme in language and aphasia: history and current state. *Cortex* 2008;44:953-961.

Cohen AL, Fair DA, Dosenbach NUF, Miezin FM, Dierker D, Van Essen DC, Schlaggar BL. Defining functional areas in individual human brains using resting functional connectivity MRI. *NeuroImage* 2008;41:45-57.

Concha ML, Bianco IH, Wilson SW. Encoding asymmetry within neural circuits. *Nature Reviews Neuroscience* 2012;13:832-843.

Corballis MC. From mouth to hand: gesture, speech, and the evolution of right-handedness. *Behavioral and Brain Sciences* 2003;26:199-260. (I also quote from Carstairs-McCarthy A. A shrug is not a sentence—which can be found on p. 215 in this citation.)

Corballis MC. Left brain, right brain: facts and fantasies. *PLoS Biology* 12(1): e1001767. doi:10.1371/journal.pbio.1001767.

Dehaene S, Cohen L, Sigman M, Vinckier F. The neural code for written words: a proposal. *Trends in Cognitive Sciences* 2005;9:335-341.

Douglas R and Martin K. Neocortex. In: *The Synaptic Organization of the Brain*. [4th ed.]. Ed. Shepherd, Gordon M. New York and Oxford: Oxford University Press, 1998, pp. 459-509.

Dronkers NF, Plaisant O, Iba-Zizen MT, Cabanis EA. Paul Broca's historic cases: high resolution MR imaging of the brains of Leborgne and Lelong. *Brain* 2007;130: 1432-1441.

Engelhardt E. Cerebrocerebellar system and Türck's bundle. *Journal of the History of the Neurosciences* 2013;22:353-365.

ffytche DH, Catani M. Beyond localization: from hodology to function. *Philosophical Transactions of the Royal Society* 2005;360:767-779.

Flechsig P. Developmental (myelogenetic) localisation of the cerebral cortex in the human subject. *Lancet* 1901;158 (issue 4077):1027-1029.

Fox MD, Raichle ME. Spontaneous fluctuations in brain activity observed with functional magnetic resonance imaging. *Nature Reviews Neuroscience* 2007;8:700-711

Geschwind N. "The work and influence of Wernicke." In: *Selected Boston Studies in the Philosophy of Science* (vol. IV), eds. Cohen, Robert S. and Wartofsky, Marx W. Dordrecht: D. Reidel Publishing, 1969, pp. 1-33.

Geschwind N. "Disconnection syndromes in animals and man." In: *Selected Papers on Language and the Brain: Boston Studies in the Philosophy of Science* (vol. XVI), eds. Cohen, Robert S. and Wartofsky, Marx W. Dordrecht and Boston: D. Reidel Publishing, 1974, pp. 106-231.

Gilden DL, Thornton T, Mallon MW. 1/f noise in human cognition. *Science* 1995;267:1837-1839.

Goldman-Rakic PS, Schwartz ML. Interdigitation of contralateral and ipsilateral columnar projections to frontal association cortex in primates. *Science* 1982;216:755-757.

Gordon EM, Laumann TO, Adeyemo B, Huckins JF, Kelley WM, Petersen SE. Generation and evaluation of a cortical area parcellation from resting-state correlations. *Cerebral Cortex* 2016;26:288-303.

Greenblatt SH. The major influences on the early life and work of John Hughlings Jackson. *Bulletin of the History of Medicine* 1965;39:346-376.

Harris LJ. Early theory and research on hemispheric specialization. *Schizophrenia Bulletin*; 1999;25:11-39.

Haymaker W, Paul Emil Flechsig. In: Haymaker W and Baer, Karl A, eds. *Founders of Neurology: One Hundred and Thirty-Three Biographical Sketches*, pp. 31-35.

Hickock G, Houde J, Rong F. Sensorimotor integration in speech processing: computational basis and neural organization. *Neuron* 2011;69:407-422.

Imaizumi K, Lee CC. Frequency transformation in the auditory lemniscal thalamocortical system. *Frontiers in Neural Circuits* 2014 (July);8:doi: 10.3389/fncir.2014.00075.

Jackson JH. On a case of loss of power of expression: inability to talk, to write, and to read correctly after convulsive attacks. *British Medical Journal* 1866;2 (Nos. 291 and 299):92-94 and 326-330.

Jackson JH. The Croonian lectures on evolution and dissolution of the nervous system. *British Medical Journal* 1884;1(No. 1213):591-593.

Jones W, Bellugi U, Lai Z, Chiles M, Reilly J, Lincoln A, Adolphs R. Hypersociability in Williams syndrome. *Journal of Cognitive Neuroscience* 2000;12 supplement 1:30-46.

Kaas JH, Hackett TA. (1999a) 'What' and 'where' processing in auditory cortex. *Nature Neuroscience* 1999;2:1045-1047.

Kaas JH, Hackett TA, Tramo MJ. (1999b) Auditory processing in primate cerebral cortex. *Current Opinion in Neurobiology* 1999;9:164-170.

Koch G, Cercignani M, Bonnì S, Giacobbe V, Bucchi G, Versace V, Caltagirone C, Bozzali M. Asymmetry of parietal interhemispheric connections in humans. *Journal of Neuroscience* 2011;31:8967-8975.

Laumann TO, Gordon EM, Adeyemo B, Snyder AZ, Joo SJ, Chen MY, Gilmore AW, McDermott KB, Nelson SM, Dosenbach NUF,

Schlaggar BL, Mumford JA, Poldrack RA, Petersen SE. Functional system and areal organization of a highly sampled individual human brain. *Neuron* 2015;87:657-670.

Margulies DS. Unraveling the complex tapestry of association networks. *Neuron* 2017;95:239-241.

Mathews PJ, Obler LK, Albert ML. Wernicke and Alzheimer on the language disturbances of dementia and aphasia. *Brain and Language* 1994;46:439-463.

Miyawaki E. C:\Evolve: [Review of Deacon T., *The Symbolic Species: The Co-Evolution of Language and the Brain* and Pinker S., *How the Mind Works*]. *The Yale Review* 1998;86(4):128-139.

Miyawaki E. By the Book. [Review of Dehaene S. *Reading in the Brain: The Science and Evolution of a Human Invention*]. *The Yale Review* 2010;98(4):140-153.

Ogawa S, Lee TM, Kay AR, Tank DW. Brain magnetic resonance imaging with contrast dependent on blood oxygenation. *Proceedings of the National Academy of Sciences* (United States) 1990;87:9868-9872.

Olry R, Haines DE. NEUROwords. Korbinian Brodmann: the Victor Hugo of cytoarchitectonic brain maps. *Journal of the History of the Neurosciences* 2010;19:195-198.

Papez JW, Theodor Meynert. In: Haymaker W and Baer, Karl A, eds. *Founders of Neurology: One Hundred and Thirty-Three Biographical Sketches.* Springfield: Charles C. Thomas, 1953, pp. 64-67.

Pickles JO. Auditory pathways. In: *Handbook of Clinical Neurology*, v. 129 (3rd series), *The Human Auditory System* [eds. Celesia GG and Hickok G]. Amsterdam: Elsevier, 2015.

Raichle ME, Mintun MA. Brain work and brain imaging. *Annual Review of Neuroscience* 2006;29:449-476.

Satterthwaite TD, Davatzikos C. Towards an individualized delineation of functional neuroanatomy. *Neuron* 2015;87:471-473.

Schmahmann JD. From movement to thought: anatomic substrate of the cerebellar contribution to cognitive processing. *Human Brain Mapping* 1996;4:174-198.

Seitelberger F. Theodor Meynert (1833-1892): Pioneer and visionary of brain research. *Journal of the History of the Neurosciences* 1997;6(3):264-274.

Shoja MM. Tubbs RS, Loukas M, Shokouhi G, Ardalan MR. Marie-François Xaxier Bichat (1771-1802) and his contributions to the foundations of pathological anatomy and modern medicine. *Annals of Anatomy* 2008;190:413-420.

Stookey B. Jean-Baptiste Bouillaud and Ernest Auburtin: early studies on cerebral localization and the speech center. *Journal of the American Medical Association* 1963;184:1024-1029.

Van Essen DC, Maunsell JHR. Two-dimensional maps of the cerebral cortex. *Journal of Comparative Neurology* 1980;191:255-281

Wernicke C. The symptom complex of aphasia. A psychological study on an anatomical basis. In: *Boston Studies in the Philosophy of Science* (vol. IV), eds. Cohen, Robert S. and Wartofsky, Marx W. Dordrecht: D. Reidel Publishing, 1969, pp. 34-97.

Whitaker HA, Etlinger SC. Theodor Meynert's contribution to classical 19th century aphasia studies. *Brain and Language* 1993;45:560-571.

Williams JCP, Barratt-Boyes BG, Lowe JB. Supravalvular aortic stenosis. *Circulation* 1961;24:1311-1318.

Yates AJ. Delayed auditory feedback. *Psychological Bulletin* 1963;60(3):213-232.

References for the Third Seminar

Books

Biousse, Valérie and Newman, Nancy J. *Neuro-ophthalmology Illustrated*. New York and Stuttgart: Thieme, 2009.

Brazis, Paul W., Masdeu, Joseph C., and Biller, José. *Localization in Clinical Neurology*. Boston and Toronto: Little, Brown, 1985.

Brodal, A. *Neurological Anatomy In Relation to Clinical Medicine*. [3rd ed.] New York and Oxford: Oxford University Press, 1981.

Carpenter, Malcolm B. and Sutin, Jerome. *Human Neuroanatomy*. [8th ed.] Baltimore and London: Williams and Wilkins, 1983.

Cordo, Paul and Harnad, Stevan, eds. *Movement Control*. New York: Cambridge University Press, 1994.

DeArmond, Stephen J., Fusco, Madeline M., and Dewey, Maynard M. *Structure of the Human Brain. A Photographic Atlas*. [3rd ed.] New York, Oxford: Oxford University Press, 1989.

Glaser, Joel S., ed. *Neuro-ophthalmology*. [2nd ed.] Philadelphia: J.B. Lippincott, 1990.

Kahle, Werner. *Nervous System and Sensory Organs*. [3rd revised ed., trans. H.L. and A.D. Dayan, Volume 3 of Kahle W., Leonhardt H, Platzer W. *Color Atlas and Textbook of Human Anatomy*] Stuttgart and New York: Georg Thieme, 1986.

Llinás, Rodolfo R. *I of the Vortex. From Neurons to Self*. Cambridge and London: MIT Press, 2001.

Nauta, Walle J.H. and Feirtag, Michael. *Fundamental Neuroanatomy*. New York: W.H. Freeman, 1986.

Nieuwenhuys, Rudolf. *Chemoarchitecture of the Brain*. Berlin/ Heidelberg/New York/Tokyo: Springer Verlag, 1985.

Nieuwenhuys, R., Voogd, J., and van Huijzen, C. *The Human Central Nervous System*. Fourth ed. Berlin/Heidelberg/New York: Springer Verlag, 2008.

Nolte, John. *The Human Brain. An Introduction to Its Functional Anatomy*. [4th ed.] St. Louis: Mosby, 1999.

Shepherd, Gordon M., ed. *The Synaptic Organization of the Brain* [4th ed]. New York and Oxford: Oxford University Press, 1998.

Swanson, Larry W. *Neuroanatomical Terminology. A Lexicon of Classical Origins and Historical Foundations*. Oxford and New York: Oxford University Press, 2015.

*

Articles and Chapters in Books

Alexander GE, DeLong MR, Crutcher MD. Naturalizing motor control theory: isn't it time for a new paradigm? In: *Movement Control*. Eds. Cordo, P and Harnard, S. Cambridge: Cambridge University Press, 1994, pp. 226-231.

Aravamuthan BR, Muthusamy KA, Stein JF, Aziz TZ, Johansen-Berg H. Topography of cortical and subcortical connections of the human pedunculopontine and subthalamic nuclei. *NeuroImage* 2007;37:694-705.

Bahsi, I, Orhan M, Kervancioglu P, Bahsi A. Constanzo Varolio (1543-1575), who named the "pons." *Child's Nervous System* 2018;34:585-588.

Baizer JS, Sherwood CC, Hof PR, Witelson SF, Sultan F. Neurochemical and structural organization of the principal nucleus of the inferior olive in the human. *The Anatomical Record* 2011;294:1198-1216.

Bisdorff AR, Wolsley CJ, Anastasopoulos D, Bronstein AM, Gresty MA. The perception of body verticality (subjective postural vertical) in peripheral and central vestibular disorders. *Brain* 1996;119:1523-1534.

Blomfield S and Marr D. How the cerebellum may be used. *Nature* 1970;227:1224-1228.

Brazis PW. The localization of lesions affecting the brainstem. In: *Localization in Clinical Neurology*. Eds. Brazis PW, Masdeu JC, Biller J. Boston and Toronto: Little, Brown, 1985, pp. 225-238.

Broga C, Fiengo L, Türe U. Achille Louis Foville's atlas of brain anatomy and Defoville syndrome. *Neurosurgery* 2012;70:1265-1273.

Bronstein AM, Pérennou DA, Guerraz M, Playford D, Rudge P. Dissociation of visual and haptic vertical in two patients with vestibular nuclear lesions. *Neurology* 2003;61:1260-1262.

Burnstock G. Autonomic neurotransmission: 60 years since Sir Henry Dale. *Annual Review of Pharmacology and Toxicology* 2009;49:1-30.

Büttner-Ennever JA. The extraocular motor nuclei: organization and functional neuroanatomy. *Progress in Brain Research* 2006;151:95-125.

Carpenter MB and Pierson RJ. Pretectal region and the pupillary light reflex. An anatomical analysis in the monkey. *Journal of Comparative Neurology* 1973;149:271-300.

Chandrasekhar A. Turning heads: development of vertebrate branchiomotor neurons. *Developmental Dynamics* 2004;229:143-161.

Chandraskehar A, Moens CB, Warren JT, Kimmel CB, Kuwada JY. Development of branchiomotor neurons in zebrafish. *Development* 1997;124:2633-2644.

Coenen VA, Schumacher LV, Kaller C, Schlaepfer TE, Reinacher PC, Egger K, Urbach H, Reisert M. The anatomy of the human medial forebrain bundle: ventral tegmental area connections to reward-associated subcortical and frontal lobe regions. *NeuroImage: Clinical* 2018;18:770-783.

Cohen B, Komatsuzaki A, Bender MB. Electrooculographic syndrome in monkeys after pontine reticular formation lesions. *Archives of Neurology* 1968;18:78-92.

Cooper ERA. The trochlear nerve in the human embryo and foetus. *British Journal of Ophthalmology* 1947;31:257-75.

Daroff RB, Troost BT, Leigh RJ. Supranuclear disorders of eye movements. In: *Neuro-ophthalmology* [2nd ed.]. Ed. Glaser JS. Philadelphia: J.B. Lippincott, 1990, pp. 299-323.'

Davidoff RA, Atkin A, Anderson PJ, Bender MB. Optokinetic nystagmus and cerebral disease. Clinical and pathological study. *Archives of Neurology* 1966;14:73-81.

Dieterich M and Brandt T. Ocular torsion and tilt of subjective vertical are sensitive brainstem signs. *Annals of Neurology* 1993;33:292-299.

Fisher CM. Ataxic hemiparesis. A pathologic study. *Archives of Neurology* 1978;35:126-128.

Fisher CM and Cole M. Homolateral ataxia and crural paresis: a vascular syndrome. *Journal of Neurology, Neurosurgery, and Psychiatry* 1965;28:48-55.

Fisher CM, Karnes WE, Kubik CS. Lateral medullary infarction–the pattern of vascular occlusion. *Journal of Neuropathology and Experimental Neurology* 1961;20:323-379.

Foville A. Note sur une paralysie peu connue de certains muscles de l'œil, et sa liaison avec quelques points de l'anatomie et la physiologie de la protubérance annulaire. *Bulletins de la Société Anatomique de Paris* 1858;33:393-414.

Fritzsch B. Of mice and genes: evolution of vertebrate brain development. *Brain, Behavior and Evolution* 1998;52:207-217.

Frohman TC, Galetta S, Fox R, Solomon D, Straumann D, Filippi M, Zee D, Frohman EM. Pearls and Oy-sters: the medial longitudinal fasciculus in ocular motor physiology. *Neurology* 2008;70:e57-e67.

Fukushima K. The interstitial nucleus of Cajal and its role in the control of movements of head and eyes. *Progress in Neurobiology* 1987;29:107-192.

Gates P. Work out where the problem is in the brainstem using 'the rule of 4.' *Practical Neurology* 2011;11:167-172.

Gautier JC and Blackwood W. Enlargement of the inferior olivary nucleus in association with lesions of the central tegmental tract or dentate nucleus. *Brain* 1961;84:341-361.

Goldman-Rakic PS. The "psychic" neuron of the cerebral cortex. *Annals of the New York Academy of Sciences* 1999;868:13-26.

Hartline PH. Physiological basis for detection of sound and vibration in snakes. *Journal of Experimental Biology* 1971;54:349-371.

Haubenberger D and Hallett M. Essential tremor. *New England Journal of Medicine* 2018;378:1802-1809.

Hikosaka O. The habenula: from stress evasion to value-based decision-making. *Nature Reviews Neuroscience* 2010;11:503-513.

Hikosaka O, Takikawa Y, Kawagoe R. Role of the basal ganglia in the control of purposive saccadic eye movements. *Physiological Reviews* 2000;80:953-978.

Hörnsten G. Wallenberg's syndrome. Part I. General symptomatology, with special reference to visual disturbances and imbalance. *Acta Neurologica Scandinavica* 1974(a);50:434-446.

Hörnsten G. Wallenberg's syndrome. Part II. Oculomotor and oculostatic disturbances. *Acta Neurologica Scandinavica* 1974(b);50:447-468.

Irving R and Harrison JM. The superior olivary complex and audition: a comparative study. *Journal of Comparative Neurology* 1967;130:77-86.

Jones EG. Golgi, Cajal and the neuron doctrine. *Journal of the History of the Neurosciences* 1999;8:170-178.

Kinney HC, Broadbelt KG, Haynes RL, Rognum IJ, Paterson DS. The serotonergic anatomy of the developing human medulla oblongata: implications for pediatric disorders of homeostasis. *Journal of Chemical Neuroanatomy* 2011;41:182-199.

Kinney HC and Samuels MA. Neuropathology of the persistent vegetative state. A review. *Journal of Neuropathology and Experimental Neurology* 1994;53:548-558.

———

Lapresle J and Hamida MB. The dentato-olivary pathway. Somatotopic relationship between the dental nucleus and the contralateral inferior olive. *Archives of Neurology* 1970;22:135-143.

Longetti P, Fiorindi A, Feletti A, D'Avella D, Martinuzzi A. Endoscopic anatomy of the fourth ventricle. Laboratory investigation. *Journal of Neurosurgery* 2008;109:530-555.

McCrea RA and Baker R. Anatomical connections of the nucleus prepositus of the cat. *Journal of Comparative Neurology* 1985;237:377-407.

McCrea RA and Horn AKE. Nucleus prepositus. *Progress in Brain Research* 2006;151:205-230.

McKay IJ, Lewis J, Lumsden A. Organization and development of facial motor neurons in the *Kreisler* mutant mouse. *European Journal of Neuroscience* 1997;9:1499-1506.

Marx JJ, Iannetti GD, Thömke F, Fitzek S, Urban PP, Stoeter P, Cruccu G, Dieterich M, Hopf HC. Somatotopic organization of the corticospinal tract in the human brainstem: a MRI-based mapping analysis. *Annals of Neurology* 2005;57:824-831.

Mastick GS and Easter SS. Initial organization of neurons and tracts in the embryonic mouse fore- and midbrain. *Developmental Biology* 1996;173:79-94.

May PJ, Reiner AJ, Ryabinin AE. Comparison of the distributions of urocortin-containing and cholinergic neurons in the perioculomotor midbrain of the cat and macaque. *Journal of Comparative Neurology* 2008;507:1300-1316.

Miyawaki EK. Cerebral Arteries. In: Aminoff MJ and Daroff RB, eds. *Encyclopedia of the Neurological Sciences* [2nd ed.]. Oxford: Academic Press, 2014, pp. 651-657.

Moore JK. The human auditory brain stem: a comparative view. *Hearing Research* 1987;29:1-32.

Moore RY and Bloom FE. Central catecholamine neuron systems: anatomy and physiology of the dopamine systems. *Annual Review of Neuroscience* 1978;1:129-169.

Moreno-Bravo JA, Martinez-Lopez JE, Puelles E. Review. Mesencephalic neuronal populations. New insights on the ventral differentiation programs. *Histology and Histopathology* 2012;27:1529-1538.

Müller F, O'Rahilly R. The development of the human brain, including the longitudinal zoning in the diencephalon at stage 15. *Anatomy and Embryology* 1988;179:55-71.

Müller F, O'Rahilly R. The initial appearance of the cranial nerves and related neuronal migration in staged human embryos. *Cells Tissues Organs* 2011;193:215-238.

Nakamura H. Regionalization of the optic tectum: combinations of gene expression that define the tectum. *Trends in Neurosciences* 2001;24:32-39.

Nathan PW and Smith MC. The rubrospinal and central tegmental tracts in man. *Brain* 1982;105:223-269.

Ngwa EC, Zeeh C, Messoudi A, Büttner-Ennever JA, Horn AKE. Delineation of motoneuron subgroups supplying individual eye muscles in the human oculomotor nucleus. *Frontiers in Neuroanatomy* 2014;8:article 2, doi: 10.3389/fnana.2014.00002.

Nieuwenhuys R. The structural, functional, and molecular organization of the brainstem. *Frontiers in Neuroanatomy* 2011;5:article 33, doi: 10.3389/fnana.2011.00033.

Ohtsuka K and Nagasaka Y. Divergent axon collaterals from the rostral superior colliculus to the pretectal accommodation-related areas and the omnipause neuron area in the cat. *Journal of Comparative Neurology* 1999;413:68-76.

Pombal MA, Megías M. Development and functional organization of the cranial nerves in lampreys. *The Anatomical Record* 2018; doi: 10.1002/ar.23821.

Puelles K, Tvrdik P, Martínez-De-La-Torre M. The postmigratory alar topography of visceral cranial nerve efferents challenges the classical model of hindbrain columns. *The Anatomical Record* 2018 Apr 16, doi: 10.1002/ar.23830.

Rakic P. A small step for the cell, a giant leap for mankind: a hypothesis of neocortical expansion during evolution. *Trends in Neurosciences* 1995;18:383-388.

Rasmussen AT and Peyton WT. Origin of the ventral external arcuate fibers and their continuity with the striae medullares of the fourth ventricle of man. *The Anatomical Record* 1946;84:325-337.

Ruigrok TJH and Voogd J. Organization of projections from the inferior olive to the cerebellar nuclei in the rat. *Journal of Comparative Neurology* 2000;426:209-228.

Salma A, Yeremeyeva E, Baidya NB, Sayers MP, Ammirati M. Neuroanatomical study. An endoscopic, cadaveric analysis of the roof of the fourth ventricle. *Journal of Clinical Neuroscience* 2013;20:710-714.

Sato T, Joyner AL, Nakamura H. Review. How does FgF signaling from the isthmic organizer induce midbrain and cerebellar development? *Development, Growth, and Differentiation* 2004;46:487-494.

Schmahmann JD, Ko R, MacMore J. The human basis pontis: motor syndromes and topographic organization. *Brain* 2004;127:1269-1291.

Selvadurai C, Rondeau MW, Colorado RA, Feske SK, Prasad S. Teaching video Neuro*Images*: Foville syndrome. *Neurology* 2016;86:e203.

Sharpe JA. What's up, doc? Altered perception of the haptic, postural, and visual vertical. *Neurology* 2003;61:1172-1173.

Shute CCD and Lewis PR. The ascending cholinergic reticular system: neocortical, olfactory and subcortical projections. *Brain* 1967;90:497-520.

Sierra-Hidalgo F, de Pablo-Fernández E, Herrero-San Martin A, Correas-Callero E, Herreros-Rodríguez J, Romero-Muñoz JP, Martín-Gil L. Clinical and imaging features of the room tilt illusion. *Journal of Neurology* 2012;259:2555-2564.

Silverman IE, Liu GT, Volpe NJ, Galetta SL. The crossed paralyses. The original brain-stem syndromes of Millard-Gubler, Foville, Weber, and Raymond-Cestan. *Archives of Neurology* 1995;52:635-638.

Sterling P. Retina. In: *The Synaptic Organization of the Brain.* Ed. Shepherd GM. New York: Oxford, 1998, see especially p. 225.

Voogd J, van Baarsen K. The horseshoe-shaped commissure of Wernekinck or the decussation of the brachium conjunctivum. Methodological changes in the 1840's. *Cerebellum* 2014;13:113-120.

Zec N, Filiano JJ, Kinney HC. Anatomic relationships of the human arcuate nucleus of the medulla; a DiI-labeling study. *Journal of Neuropathology and Experimental Neurology* 1997;56:509-522.